Laminitis & Founder

Prevention and Treatment for the Greatest Chance of Success

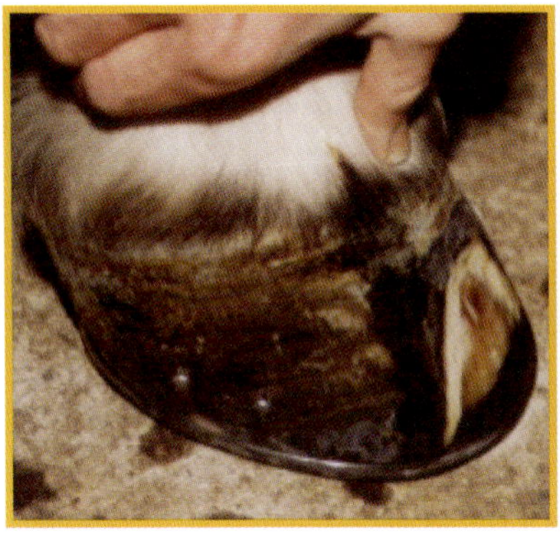

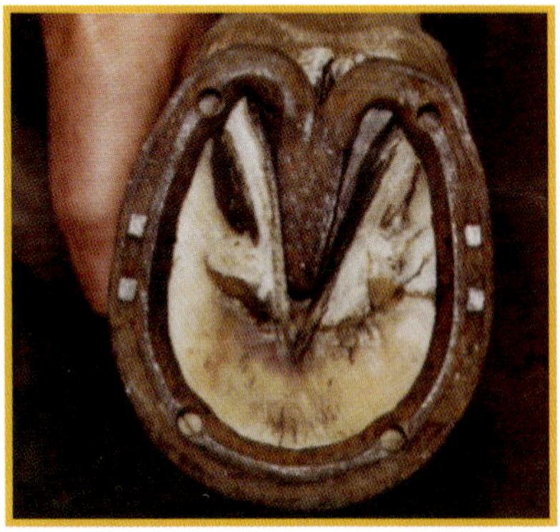

featuring
The Edema Theory
The Frog Support Theory

By Doug Butler, PhD, CJF, FWCF
and Frank Gravlee, DVM, MS, CNS

Book designed and edited by:
Carr Creative, Fort Collins, Colorado

Published by:
Life Data Labs, Inc.
12290 Hwy. 72
Cherokee, Alabama 35616
1-256-370-7555

ISBN: 978-0-9794857-0-1

Additional resources available at:
www.dougbutler.com
www.lifedatalabs.com

Table of Contents

"We dedicate this work to all the horses that have lost their lives to these devastating diseases."

Introduction

There are many myths and half-truths surrounding laminitis and founder. Our purpose is to present a practical, yet credible, guide for modern horse owners. While we acknowledge the significant work of other equine scientists and practitioners on laminitis and founder, many ideas presented here are the result of our own personal research and experience.

Our desire is to help horse owners make informed decisions. Some popular and currently held theories on the causes and treatments of laminitis and founder are at odds with what we present. However, we hope you will consider our professional credibility and successful experiences in trying and testing these techniques. We present the facts as we understand them, and believe them to be sound.

This book identifies swelling (edema) of the laminar tissues and sublaminar tissues as a cause of laminitis and founder. We will discuss select treatments and procedures. Laminitis and founder are often components or symptoms of another disease or condition which must be treated concurrently or simultaneously. Each case must be considered individually. These discussions should not be interpreted as medical advice. Accordingly, we recommend that you consult with your veterinarian/farrier team regarding the health and care of your horse.

In order to have the greatest chance for a successful outcome, the horse owner must become the equine professional's ally when treating laminitis and founder. We hope this information will help farriers, veterinarians and horse owners work together for the good of the horse. Ultimately, the horse owner must make the final decision as to what is best for the horse.

It is important for horse owners to understand the severity of laminitis and founder, and to see how important it is to use sound, time-tested mechanical, as well as medical, treatment regimens. Horses treated with more attention to detail have a greater chance of recovery. We have successfully treated many animals severely affected by these diseases. However, you must realize that some horses will not recover — no matter how treated.

Studies confirm laminitis is a serious problem

The seriousness of the laminitis problem in the United States can be seen in the results of the 1998 National Animal Health Monitoring System Equine Study by the USDA-APHIS, which reflected these statistics:

74% Recovered
12% Showed no improvement, only got worse
8% Improved, but remained lame
6% Died, naturally or were euthanized

Another study a few years ago at Cornell University estimated that 1-1/2 percent of America's horse population is affected each year by laminitis (about 100,000 cases). A study in the United Kingdom determined that about 3 percent of the horses there are affected (about 20,000 cases). In Canada, the

University of Guelph determined by survey that laminitis is the No. 1 equine health concern to horse owners. Yet, it appears that little progress has been made in the prevention and treatment of laminitis in the past 100 years.

Today there is an abundance of divergent information concerning laminitis. However, the lack of reliable information on laminitis and founder has resulted in an apparent increase in the incidence and severity of these diseases.

We believe horse owners should be well informed before making decisions concerning the welfare of their horses. A good decision can make the difference between a horse living or dying. It is our goal to provide you with the most reliable information based on our education and experience with clinical cases to assist you in making those informed decisions.

In order to choose the most effective treatment regimen for laminitis and founder, the caregivers must understand the predisposing cause, stage of the disease, mode of action and how best to prevent future attacks. The cause must be determined and subsequently removed or neutralized. This book emphasizes that the swelling must be reduced to prevent further damage to the sensitive foot tissues; that the damaged structures must be supported so the body can repair them; and, finally, that the destroyed tissue must be rebuilt by feeding the horse a balanced diet that includes nutrients that support dermal tissues.

1

Defining Equine Laminitis and Founder

What is equine laminitis?

Laminitis is a serious disease or condition that affects the laminae of the horse's foot. The laminae are Velcro-like projections that attach the hoof to the coffin bone, or distal phalanx (DP), contained within the foot. Laminitis may affect one foot, the front feet only, the hind feet only or all four feet.

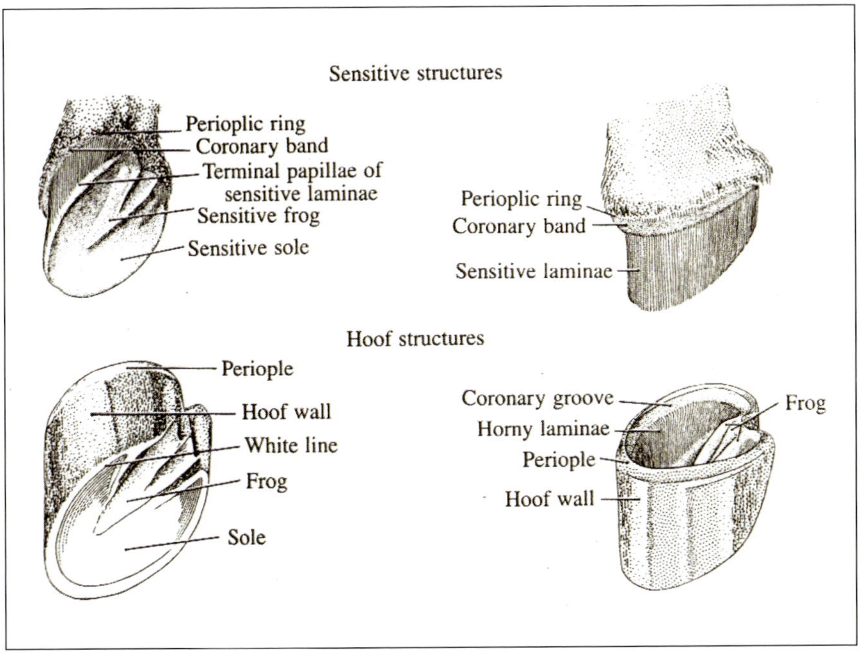

Figure 1-1. *The sensitive structures are the source of growth and nournishment of the hoof structures. Drawings by L. Sadler.*

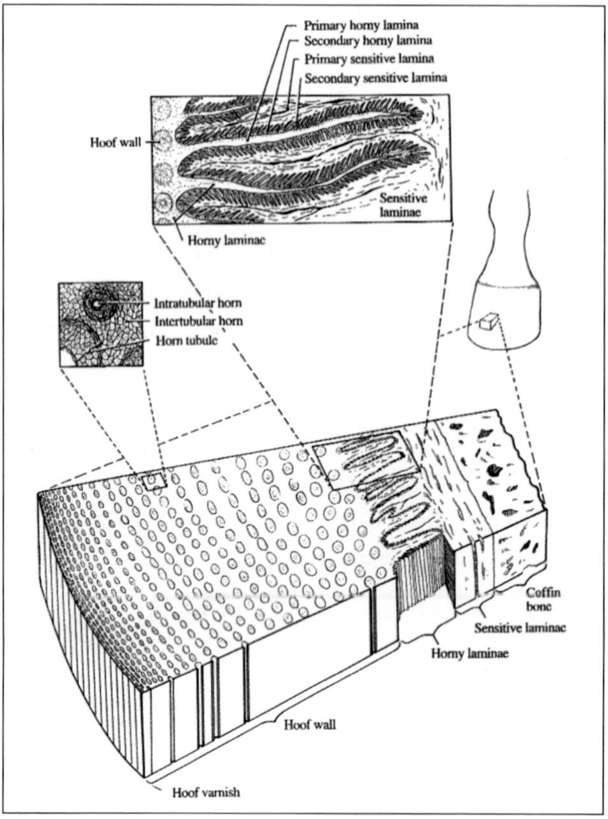

Figure 1-2. *Wall structure and hoof/bone bond. Drawings by L. Sadler. © 2004 Doug Butler Enterprises, Inc. Used by permission.*

The word laminitis implies that the laminar tissues are inflamed. Fluids have moved from the affected blood vessels into the interstitial tissue, creating pressure between the two solid bodies of hoof and bone. The pressure from the swollen tissues surrounding the nerves causes intense pain.

As a result of swelling, the tissues in the foot, including laminae, subdermal connective tissue (collagen fibrils) and periosteal (outer bone covering) structures are compressed in the closed space (vault) between the hoof and coffin bone. The pressure on the nerves and blood vessels in the sensitive laminar and sole tissue causes great pain and suffering. The horse may be unable to stand comfortably within a few hours after onset.

A significant amount of space is occupied by the lumen of normal blood vessels in the foot. The swelling is a result of fluid moving from inside the blood vessels into the tissues surrounding the vessels. The rising fluid pressure outside the blood vessels in the tissues trapped between the coffin bone and hoof capsule causes the blood vessels to collapse, gradually cutting off the blood flow.

Organ tissues in the body have varying capacities for maintaining normal activity during stress. A certain percentage of healthy tissue is needed to maintain normal activity without producing disease symptoms. For example, the kidneys and lungs have enough capacity to maintain normal function (producing no symptoms) even when 50 percent or more of their function is lost due to disease.

The horse's circulation capacity in the foot is in excess of what is needed for normal and even strenuous activity. Horses typically do not show signs of laminitis until a significant amount of laminar tissue is damaged. However, previous episodes of laminitis result in compromised tissue, requiring less of an insult to reach the trigger point where symptoms of laminitis disease become evident. Again, the scar tissue won't absorb as much pressure and will tear rather than stretch. This explains why it is easier for the horse to develop laminitis with each successive insult to this tissue.

The laminar scarring progresses along a timeline through a sequence of events, gradually becoming more serious. For this reason, it is a medical emergency to restore circulation by

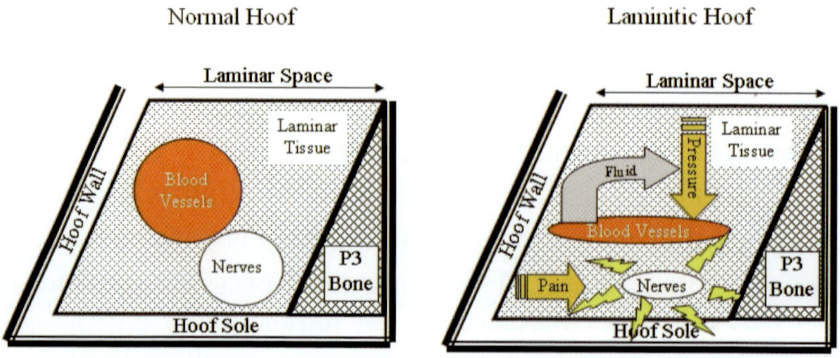

In the normal hoof, the fluid within the blood vessel is in osmotic equilibrium with the surrounding tissue. Fluid moves from within the blood vessel into the laminar tissue at the same rate that fluid moves back into the blood vessel. The blood vessels are fully open for optimum circulation of blood.

In the laminitic hoof, more fluid is moving out of the blood vessels than is moving into them. The result is increased pressure in the closed laminar space causing vascular collapse, intense pain and tissue necrosis.

Figure 1-3. *Diagramatic illustration of the effect of fluid leaking into the interstitial tissues. Provided by Life Data Labs Research Farms.*

reducing the edema before anoxia (lack of oxygen) occurs, therefore preventing damage. Once necrosis (tissue death) occurs due to anoxia, the time to prevent and/or reverse the disease process has passed.

As the disease progresses, the laminar junction between the coffin bone and hoof is destroyed due to compromised circulation, and the fluid pressure pushes the hoof capsule away from the bone (called rotation) causing a deformed hoof. The combination of pressure from within the hoof pushing out and the horse's body weight pushing down causes the bone to eventually founder (called sinking).

Due to pressure necrosis, laminitis usually progresses from inflammation at a cellular level to tissue destruction. The horny and sensitive laminar junction separates, and the horse becomes physically foundered when the relationship between the hoof and bone changes.

The object is to recognize and treat laminitis early — before it moves to the more destructive founder.

What is founder?

Founder is a nautical term meaning "sink." The rotation or sinking of the bone in the hoof is the result of the swollen tissue pushing the hoof apart from the bone and the horse's body weight pulling the bone and hoof apart due to the weakened laminar connection.

Horses can be affected mildly or severely. There may be mild inflammation in the foot, or there may be widespread tissue death with the hoof becoming so distorted and/or the bone column sinking so far that the coffin bone may perforate the sole. When this occurs, the risk of becoming refractory (resistant) to treatment and progressing to a fatal bone infection called osteomyelitis is increased.

The hoof capsule can rotate and the bone column can sink (called capsular rotation) with the phalanges remaining in line. Or the coffin bone can rotate at the coffin joint (called phalangeal rotation) due to contraction of the deep flexor muscles caused by foot pain and/or the continued heel growth and compromised toe growth from compression of blood vessels in the anterior of the coronary band region. The compression of the coronary band is a result of upward pressure from the hoof wall. Along with the foundering in the feet, other tissues confined in a vault such as the teeth, kidneys and brain, are often affected. The same process is occurring — increasing fluid pressure in a confined space.

2

A Brief History and Perspective on Laminitis and Founder

After watching a mid-19th century wagon train reenactment, we asked a participating veterinarian, "What was the most important lesson you learned from the experience?" He said: "I learned just how dependent the pioneers were upon their animals. They took care of them first every morning and every evening before they fed themselves."

Things have changed a lot since the horse-and-buggy days, and as a society we don't have that same sensitivity and dependence on horses today that people previously had. It is often difficult for us to totally understand the importance of the horse in generations past; however, laminitis has always been a significant problem. Nearly every book about horses from the earliest times references these terrible diseases and their impact on human lives. For example:

Dr. E. Wilcox (*Agr. Hist.* 18:105, 1944.) stated that Custer's cavalry massacre at Little Big Horn was partially due to laminitis caused by selenium toxicity. Major Reno's troops carrying supplies and ammunition did not reach Custer in time because the pack train was slow, traveling only 10 miles a day instead of the expected 30. Many of the horses and mules were lame. The army was short of hay and wintered their animals in an area with seleniferous soils and plants. The horses belonging to the Indians led by Sitting Bull were wintered outside the seleniferous area. It wasn't until the 1930s that selenium was identified as a toxic element that causes laminitis and founder.

The teaching often determines the principles

The many divergent views among horse professionals about laminitis is caused by following inadequately proven hypotheses. If a hypothesis consistently fails, it should be questioned. For instance, what principles of laminitis and founder prevention and therapy have worked with some degree of consistency? What makes sense?

A prevalent theory taught to veterinarian and farrier students today is that laminitis is caused by vasoconstriction, therefore, the treatment should be vasodilation. This is a clinically unproven theory that was formally adopted in the early 1980s (Proceedings First Equine Endotoxemia-Laminitis Symposium – *AAEP Newsletter* 2, June, 1982). This theory reversed the ideas that were mainstream before that time. The lack of progress for 25 years is a result of abandoning sound conventional wisdom. New research dictates that we severely question the vasodilation theory.

As a community of horse owners, it appears we don't know as much about preventing or curing laminitis now as people did years ago. Books written when horses were the principal means of transportation and farm power, even those from 100 years ago, were often more accurate than some of the confusing information available today. Practitioners and horse foot specialists of that time saw many more cases of laminitis in their daily practice, and most horse owners were much more dependent and intimately involved with their animals than we are today. Because their livelihood depended on the horse's health, only the most effective treatments survived.

Foot circulation and the mechanics of the disease process were also better understood at that time. The cause and successful treatments for laminitis were often better explained by those earlier writings.

The number of horses and their economic impact declined rapidly after World War II, reaching an all-time low in 1960. Funding for equine research became almost non-existent. Expertise in horses disappeared from veterinary colleges. Farriers almost became extinct, and there was no incentive for young people to learn the trade from the "old masters." Horses became a hobby instead of a livelihood.

Fortunately, a few pockets of horse activity prevented extinction. Horses were preserved by the romance of cowboy movies, the competition of sport horses in the Olympics and racing, and the working of farms and logging with draft horses by traditionalist groups. But much knowledge was lost in the meantime.

More specialized training and research is needed

Today we live in a society that lacks intuitive understanding of the horse and its unique problems. After the horse's role as a transportation and work animal diminished, research funding dried up. An understanding of the anatomy and mechanics of the horse's foot was all but lost. The horse was replaced by the dog as the species of reference in veterinary schools. Today, many who have become competent in horse foot care have been successful due to individual effort.

Without the solid data from species-specific research, some scientists have tried to apply research from other species to the horse. For this to be successful there must be a thorough understanding of the similarities and differences in physiology and anatomy between the different species. As one prominent animal scientist said: "Data has little value unless they are applied to the species they are collected from. Data from one sheep is better than that from a hundred rats, if that data is to be applied to sheep." (McCay, C.M. *Notes on the History of Nutrition Research*, edited by F. Verzar. Hans Huber. Berne, 1973.)

We must pay more attention to the uniqueness of the horse if we desire to make progress in its care; specifically, more research on the horse's foot is desperately needed. Veterinary schools need to offer more opportunity for specialization in equine medicine, surgery and nutrition. Higher standards for admission and teaching of farrier skills must be adopted for all farrier-related programs.

Until these changes occur, we must rely on our personal clinical experience (and that of other respected horse foot care experts) as our best source of knowledge. And while we may have had many years of formal education, it is our past, present and future clinical experience that teaches us what works and what doesn't.

Incorrect teachings have caused much unnecessary suffering

The acceptance of unproven theories about laminitis has had a negative effect upon recovery of many horses. Three examples of unproven teachings introduced in the last 40 years are: 1) the theory that all hoof growth originates at the coronary band; 2) the theory on the need for vasodilation in acute laminitis; and 3) the theory of using heat therapy on the feet (hot water soaks) as a treatment for laminitis.

1) Prior to 1967, farrier and veterinary textbooks stated that the exterior hoof wall developed from the coronary band and that the interior hoof wall, or horny laminae, was produced by the sensitive laminae of the interior hoof wall. Dr. J. Stump of Indiana did some of the first electron microscopy studies on the horse's foot. After looking at sections of the coronary band, he concluded that the entire hoof wall, including the horny laminae, was produced at the coronary band (Stump, J. E. *J. of Amer. Vet. Med. Assoc.* 151:1588, 1967).

Since that time, further research has shown that this information was incomplete. Studies in Scotland by S. Kempson and in Australia by C. Pollitt using radioactive markers have shown that 20 to 30 percent of the lower hoof wall comes from the sensitive laminae of the inner hoof wall. We know this is true because the hoof wall is a cone that is larger at the base than at the top, while maintaining its thickness. The additional hoof wall at the bottom is produced by outward growth from the sensitive laminae, adding thickness to the hoof wall as the hoof grows down from the coronary band. Thus, nutrition can make a difference throughout the internal hoof wall in a few weeks rather than the eight months to one year that we previously had believed was necessary.

2) Another example is the idea that developed from the correct observation that blood is restricted in a laminitic foot. The proposed idea was that if the blood vessels are dilated, fluid can pass on through. This idea was almost universally adopted. However, since the vessels are enclosed in a vault between the hoof and bone, this idea ignores the fact that the vessels are collapsing from pressure outside the vessels. Relaxing the muscle walls of the vessels only makes the

situation worse. Recent studies verify that vasodilators such as nitroglycerine do not increase circulation in a laminitic foot.

3) The third example is the use of hot water foot soaks to replace the traditional treatment for laminitis of standing a horse in cold water, such as a stream. Only in recent years have researchers reversed the position of soaking the foot in hot water taken some 40 years ago. Now, some researchers correctly recommend cold water soaks at the first sign of laminitis. Cold water constricts the vessels, which reduces fluid leakage into the tissues, resulting in less swelling.

Because of their sincere desire to help the horse, many equine care providers have accepted erroneous information, fad shoes and unproven techniques to treat laminitis. Many more laminitic horses could have recovered if trimmed and shod using traditional and proven principles. The acceptance of fads is the result of clever marketing and deceptive promotion rather than solid research — and must be avoided at all cost. Properly trimming and shoeing a laminitic horse can be a very challenging and difficult task but after it is finished the horse will be the first to thank the farrier.

The foot must be understood before effective treatments will be adopted

Once there is a more thorough understanding of the anatomy of the foot and the sequence of events in the disease process, effective treatments for laminitis will be adopted. Ineffective fads or unproven treatments will then be discarded because of inconsistent results that also can be dangerous to the health of the horse.

For instance, giving a horse phenylbutazone (Bute) so that it continues to stand and walk on the injured laminar and solar tissues is contraindicated (not advisable). Also, vasodilators will not open crushed blood vessels. Vasodilators will cause the vascular muscle walls to relax and the vessels will actually leak more fluid into the interstitial space to further crush them. Giving a horse anti-histamine and vasoconstrictor drugs is more logical.

Another example: Standing a horse in sand, on foam blocks or putting on a "sole pack" to support the bone is not advisable. If you understand the blood supply of the foot, you will readily see that the sensitive sole will be further damaged by having the horse stand with pressure on the sole. However, transferring weight from the damaged sensitive laminae to the frog using a heart bar shoe is recommended, as there is much less circulation in the tissues under the frog than in those under the sole.

A farrier with knowledge of laminitis and the anatomy of the foot understands how to make and fit a heart bar shoe. A veterinarian with knowledge of anatomy and circulation of the foot will understand not to give pain relievers if this encourages the laminitic horse to remain standing and produce further damage to the internal structures of the foot by compromising circulation to the coffin bone *(The Principles of Horseshoeing - P3)*. When this happens you may swap a few hours of pain relief for a lifetime of lameness and pain.

This is a difficult decision because of the veterinarian's emotional and professional responsibility to relieve pain. However, the most effective pain relief is for the horse to lie down in deep bedding. This not only avoids the side effects of pain relief medications, but also facilitates the application of cold packs.

Trust yourself to learn and understand what is best for your unique horse. You have the responsibility to choose the best possible care and make crucial informed decisions for your horse(s) — use it wisely. The informed horse owner can help make decisions with trusted professionals to provide the horse with the greatest chance of getting well.

Popular theories for the cause and treatment of laminitis

Over the years there have been many theories proposed to explain laminitis. The most popular ones are presented here. And while each seems to have some merit, only the edema theory best explains what is happening.

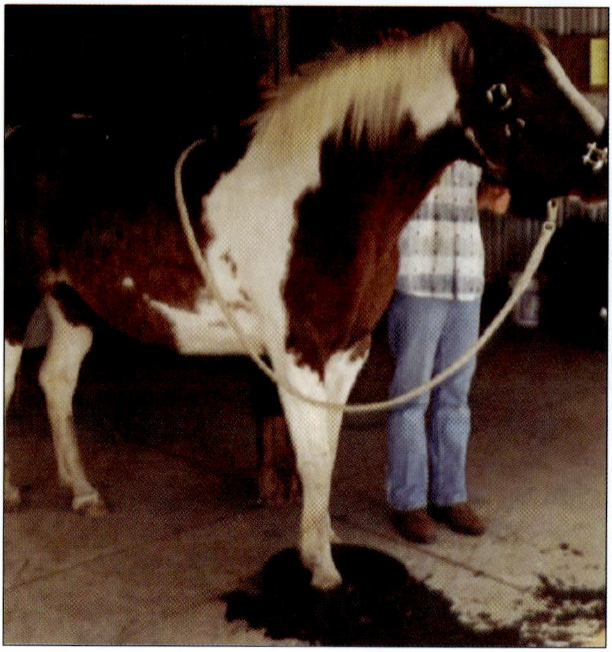

Figure 2-1. *Soak the feet in cold water when laminitis is first suspected. Soak the feet in hot water with Epsom salts to draw out foot abscesses. Photo © 2004 Doug Butler Enterprises, Inc. Used by permission.*

Inflammation theory. This was the original theory about laminitis and the one that gave the disease its name. The "itis" part of the word means inflammation. Although the chemistry and physiology of the disease were not then understood, it did explain the swelling of the tissues and resulting tissue death quite well.

Keratinization theory. This theory was introduced in the late 1940s and early 1950s and suggests that the altered metabolism of hoof keratinization at the origin of hoof growth results in a change in the sulfur content of hooves, which results in a weakening of hoof tubules and dorsal deformation of the hoof wall. This theory does not adequately explain the development of laminitis.

Enterotoxemia theory. This theory was popular in the late 1970s and early 1980s. In this theory, toxins such as moldy feed, black walnut shavings and selenium poisoning were implicated. A vaccine and anti-toxin were developed and marketed but proved ineffective in treating cases of laminitis that were not of endotoxemic origin.

Shunt theory. This theory was introduced in the late 1980s. The arteriovenous anastomosis (AVA) shunts in the extremities normally open and close to regulate body temperature in warm-blooded animals, helping to maintain a constant temperature in the body's vital central core. This system was thought to go awry in laminitis, preventing blood from returning to the laminar tissues of the foot. It was theorized this was a mechanism causing the lack of blood supply leading to necrosis or tissue death.

Enzymatic theory. This theory was introduced in the late 1990s. Metalloproteinase enzymes that are normally

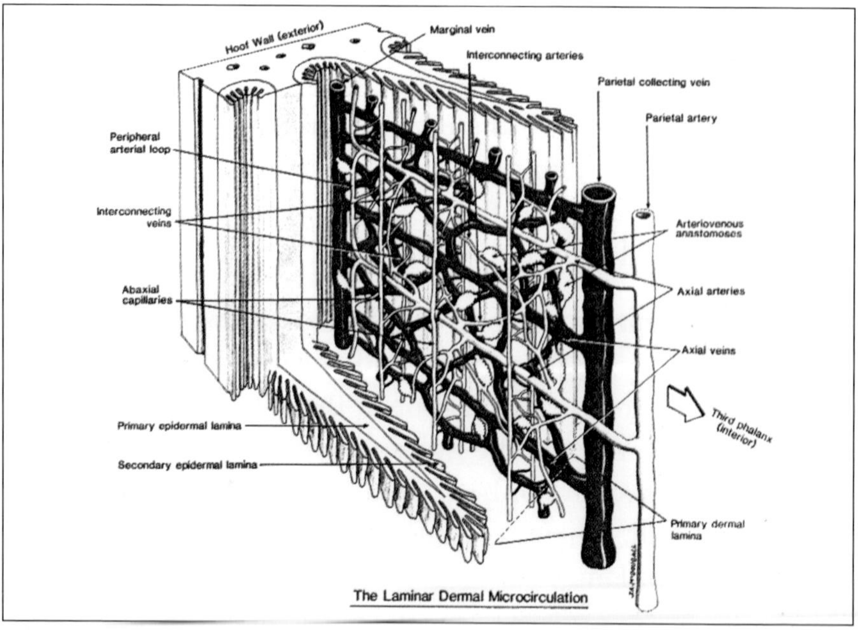

Figure 2-2. *Diagram of microcirculation of a primary dermal lamina. Drawing by J. McDougall from Pollitt and Molyneux (1990).*

released when cells are near death were thought to be the cause of laminitis by affecting the integrity of the basement membrane between the sensitive and horny laminae. Virginiamycin was used to block the production of these enzymes but was ineffective after signs of laminitis appeared.

Vasoconstriction theory. This theory has been promoted since the mid 1960s and accepted since the early 1980s. The use of vasodialator drugs, such as nitroglycerine, isoxsuprine and acepromazine, are administered to increase blood flow by relaxing the smooth muscle of blood vessels. However, these drugs are of questionable value as they cannot improve blood flow through a collapsed vessel. In addition, they increase vessel leakage in the gut and foot, as do steroids, creating more pressure in the space between hoof and bone, which in turn creates more swelling and pain. Heparin (or Warfarin) has been prescribed to thin the blood, but we don't recommend its use because it can result in internal bleeding.

Hormone theory. This theory is often referred to as equine metabolic syndrome or carbohydrate overload, and blames increases in the body's hormone production of cortisol and insulin as the cause of laminitis, especially in older horses. This theory has gained in popularity since the mid 1990s. Pergolide mesylate (Permax), prescribed in the treatment of Cushing's disease, prevents the adrenal gland from producing cortisol by suppressing the ACTH (adrenocorticotropic hormone) producing cells of the pituitary gland. Pergolide also lowers the horse's immunity, which may make them even more susceptible to laminitis.

Pain theory. Popular for the last 50 years, this theory blames the tissue death and the initial rotation of the coffin bone on the pain of laminitis. Deep flexor muscle contracture is said to cause the pain rather than a more likely possibility that it results from pain. Since the 1970s, Bute (phenylbutazone) has been promoted as the treatment for laminitis in an effort to control cellulitis and pain. Prostoglandin inhibitors such as phenylbutazone (Bute) and flunixin megalumine (Banamine) are not effective for long-term use and are ineffective for the treatment of laminitis. If you relieve the horse's pain, it continues to stand and move, further damaging the laminar connection. Eventually the coffin bone is damaged and may become infected. Bute has a negative effect on healing, may cause ulceration of the stomach and may inhibit thyroid gland function. In addition, long-term administration of Bute suppresses the metabolism of cartilage cells and makes them more susceptible to damage (Beluch,

Bertone, Anderson and Rohde. *Amer. J. Vet. Research*. 62:1916-1921, 2001).

Edema theory. As presented in this book, the edema theory states that the swelling of the laminar and sublaminar tissue is caused by various physical (from the body), psychological (from the mind) and pathological (from disease) processes resulting from excess cortisol or other conditions resulting in fluid retention. This theory is the most credible since all cases of laminitis, regardless of inciting cause, result in an edema problem. Edema is defined as an abnormally large amount of fluid in the intercellular (interstitial) spaces of the body tissues. Pressure from this fluid prevents blood from passing through the vessels, and nutrient-starved tissues die.

Since success is conditional upon choice of treatment, correct theory selection becomes essential to increasing the rate of success in treating laminitis and founder.

3

Causes of Laminitis

There are many different disease processes and conditions that can promote edema, resulting in fluid moving out of the blood vessels into the tissues. Some examples are as follows:

1) A molar imbalance between the blood vessels and tissues can result from excess salt (sodium) intake or retention, excess sugar (glucose) intake or retention in the tissues due to insulin resistance or deficiency, or deficiency of protein in the blood. Molar imbalance creates osmosis, which means that

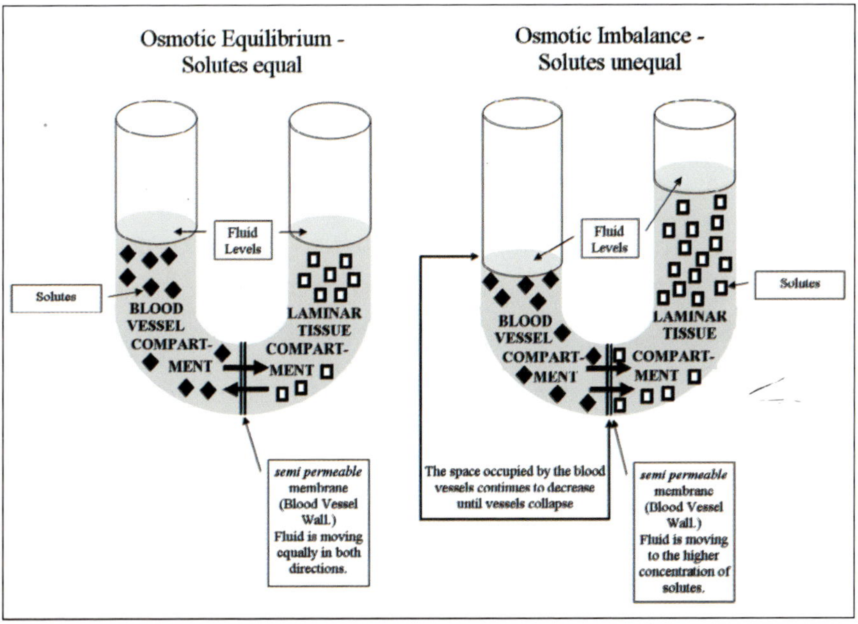

Figure 3-1. *Osmosis. Provided by Life Data Labs Equine Nutrition Research Farm.*

water flows in response to the concentration or molarity of the solutes on either side of a semi-permeable membrane or vascular wall. Water flows toward the side of greatest concentration of sugar, protein or salt.

2) Systemic toxins due to enterotoxemia (poisons in the blood coming from the gut) and septicemia (infection in the blood) lead to leaky blood vessel walls by attacking and weakening the endothelial cells that line the blood vessels.

3) Relaxation of the smooth muscle of the blood vessel walls (vasodilation) and subsequent stretching of blood vessel walls allows the blood vessels to become leaky. Vasodilators may be produced by microbes in the gut, laminar blood vessels, or they may be administered via drugs such as nitroglycerine and isoxsuprine.

4) Trauma to laminar and solar corium vessels can result from road concussion, coffin bone fracture, poor farriery including sole pressure called "sole support," or not dressing back the distorted wall at the toe, as well as compensatory lameness when the opposite limb is injured.

5) Compromised circulation due to failure to move blood through the vessels can result from congestive heart failure, anemia, shock, pressure bandages or casts.

The edema theory

There are a multitude of diseases, conditions or occurrences that can result in edema (swelling) within the hoof (unyielding and coffin-like) that can cause laminitis. The severity of laminitis symptoms is determined by the amount of pressure created inside the hoof vault by the edema and the amount of time the pressure is present. When the pressure is of enough magnitude and persists over enough time, it will create necrosis (tissue death) that leads to founder. A study of laminitis should include the causes, treatments and prevention of all diseases and conditions that have lower limb swelling of the equine as a component. Table 1 (below) illustrates examples of conditions that create edema.

Table 1. Causes of Laminitis Related to the Mechanisms Creating Edema

Conditions Having Laminitis as a Component	Mechanisms Creating Edema				
	Changes in Molarity (Osmosis)				Mechanical
	Increase Tissue Molarity = Edema		Decrease Blood Molarity = Edema		Damage to Tissue and Blood Vessels
	Tissue Sodium Increased	Tissue Protein or Sugar Increased	Blood Sodium Decreased	Blood Protein Decreased	Release of Destructive Enzymes, Serum, and/or Blood Cells into Laminar Tissue
Dietary					
Colic		+			+
Fructans		+			
Diarrhea	+				
Starvation				+	
Excess Calories		+			
During Growth					
Toxins					
Black walnut					+
Salt excess	+				
Infections					
Septicemia					+
Endocrine					
Hypothyroid		+			
Metabolic syndrome (Increased Corticoids)	+	?			
Cushing's disease	+				
Insulin resistance		+ (inter-cellular)			
Mechanical					
Road foun der					+
Off loading body weight due to injuries					+
Trauma to foot					+
Standing long time					+
Unskilled farrier					+
Stress					
Emotional	+				
Pain	+				
Toxic	+				

The mechanism creating the edema dictates the treatment of the edema — regardless of any disease processes that lead to the edema. The edema is a symptom. For example: An excess of adrenal hormone can lead to edema. We treat the edema by limiting sodium intake, increasing sodium excretion and increasing potassium intake. The adrenal disease is treated separately by administering the latest adrenal regulation medications. In the case of colic, we treat the edema by attempting to stop fluid leakage from the damaged blood vessels by administering vasoconstrictors, ice packs, etc. The colic is treated separately. In other words, treat the edema as an emergency and treat the *cause* of the edema as a separate problem.

Conditions that have laminitis as a component

The conditions that can have equine laminitis and founder as a component are divided into six categories: dietary, toxins, infections, endocrine or hormonal, mechanical and stress (see Table 1 on page 25). Several of these may be grouped into one general and popular term: equine metabolic syndrome.

1. Dietary

- Acute indigestion producing colic and/or diarrhea from overeating carbohydrates (sugars and starches in grains or sugars, starches and fructans in grasses).
- Chronic obesity from over-consumption of sugars, starches and fructans.
- Diet deficiency in essential nutrients such as protein, copper or zinc.

- Energy excess that causes rapid growth resulting in club foot (as a weanling) or knuckling over (as a yearling). (Hintz, H.F. *AAEP Proceedings.* 24:455-459, 1978).

2. Toxins

- Salt excess caused by biting off chunks from salt blocks or excess salt added to the feed.
- Toxemia (toxins in the blood) from poisons such as juglone in black walnut shavings or the enterotoxins produced by colic.

3. Infections

- Septicemia (infection in the blood) such as postpartum metritis due to retained placenta (foal founder).
- Systemic illness (usually a gram-negative bacterial disease with a fever).

4. Endocrine (Hormonal)

- Hypothyroidism with slowing metabolism resulting in weight gain and fat deposits over the eyes.
- Cushing's disease is usually the result of a pituitary tumor, and can also cause a thick neck crest, pot belly, fat rolls over the loin, swollen sheath, retained long hair, sweating and increased water consumption.
- The administration of drugs, especially the corticosteroids such as dexamethasone, can create endocrine imbalances.
- Insulin resistance interferes with carbohydrate metabolism of the laminar tissue, with high insulin levels also shown to be a vascular dilator. Could the vasodilator effect

contribute to the laminitis often associated with metabolic syndrome?

5. **Mechanical**

- Genetic predisposition to club foot and/or weak laminar attachment, especially in some bloodlines of Arabians and Morgans, small-footed Quarter Horses, weak-footed Thoroughbreds and Warm Bloods. (Club foot can also be acquired by over-nutrition as a foal.)
- Once a horse has developed laminitis, the laminae are weakened due to scar tissue formation. Each successive episode of laminitis lowers the threshold for the next bout.
- Laminar damage can be caused by repeated over-exertion and bruising of the laminar corium on hard roads at speed.
- Trauma to the foot or the animal can result in edema of the laminae.
- Standing still in a stall, trailer or ship for a long time can result in laminar edema.
- Compensatory laminitis often occurs opposite of an injured limb.
- Unskilled farriery can result in laminitis.

6. **Stress**

- A sudden change in diet or irregularity in feeding routine.
- Digestive upset or parasite infestation causing colic.
- Being separated from a favorite companion.
- Exposure to severe stormy weather.
- Sudden change in body temperature due to change in weather or illness.

Table 2. The Interaction of the Thyroid and Adrenal Gland with each other and with the Nutrients Tyrosine and Selenium.*

	Blood Serum T3 (RIA)	Blood Serum Cortisol
Blood Serum T3 (RIA)		-0.33329** (45 visits)
Blood Serum Tyrosine	+0.34689** (62 visits)	-0.10888** (43 visits)
Blood Serum Selenium	-0.45446** (59 visits)	+0.54440** (42 visits)

* These previously unpublished data are from a data bank of over 300 horses collected by Dr. Gravlee between 1978 and 2005. Each horse had a varying number of visits. The blood samples were subjected to numerous tests – some having as many as 200 analyses. To establish a correlation between two variables, both tests must be done using the same sample (visit). Only five of the hundreds (if not thousands) of nutritional correlations possible from this data are listed in the table above. The horses were Thoroughbreds and Arabians of all ages and activities. The horses were in good health and condition. The samples were taken between 7:00 a.m. and 12:00 noon. They were frozen and shipped on dry ice when indicated and the tests were performed by certified clinical laboratories.

** Correlation coefficients or r values (+ indicates a positive correlation, - indicates a negative correlation).

Equine metabolic syndrome

The metabolic interactions of nutrients and hormones must be understood if progress is to be made in the diagnosis, treatment and prevention of laminitis and founder. The genetics of the horse regulates its basic physiology. The term "easy keeper" has been used for centuries to refer to horses that get fat on very little feed. Many times laminitis and founder are associated with easy keepers that are fed excess calories resulting in metabolic syndrome problems.

Why is the easy keeper (metabolic syndrome) more susceptible to laminitis? The basal metabolic rate is controlled by the thyroid hormone. The result of low iodine, low tyrosine and/or high selenium is low thyroid output. Low thyroid hormone levels create high cortisol output, causing increased tissue sodium retention, thereby producing laminar edema and vascular compression, which causes laminitis and founder.

Excess cortisol production, insulin resistance and excess carbohydrate intake are generally accepted to be components of equine metabolic syndrome.

Dr. F. Gravlee began collecting equine nutritional and clinical data on the relationship between nutrients and healthy tissues in 1976. Table 2 on page 29 illustrates some of the interactions observed. These data establish that, as has been recently published for other species, there is a negative correlation between T3 (thyroid hormone) and cortisol, while there is a very strong, positive correlation between T3 and the amino-acid tyrosine. Tyrosine must be present for the thyroid gland to manufacture thyroxin. Tyrosine has a negative effect on cortisol production. This illustrates the profound influence of nutrients on hormones and, therefore, metabolism.

Based on this information, tyrosine was supplemented to T3 deficient horses with remarkable results (unpublished data). These research data, combined with the knowledge that tyrosine is a necessary building block for thyroid hormone, dictated the addition of tyrosine to the original Farrier's Formula®.

The antioxidant selenium has a strong negative relation to T3 and a strong positive relation to cortisol (See Table 2 on page 29). Is it possible that the popularity of selenium supplementation has resulted in over-supplementation of selenium and contributed to the epidemic of metabolic syndrome?

The above information demonstrates the importance of basing our nutrition decisions on real numbers collected from real horses. It is more logical to treat nutrition problems with nutrition management than to use drugs such as pergolide (Permax). Drugs should only be used when absolutely necessary.

Horses that are at risk for laminitis should have a blood test. A refractive index test to determine the molarity of the blood plasma can be performed in the field by the veterinarian using a hand-held refractometer. More complex laboratory tests could include ACTH, cortisol, glucose, insulin and trigicerides. These levels should be measured when the horse is calm.

A complete blood count, or CBC 20, is a bank of twenty tests including a white blood cell count. If the white blood cell count is elevated, it can indicate infection, or, if the white blood cell count is depressed, or lower, it can indicate immunity is low. A metabolic blood profile is a commercial bank of tests that includes chemical markers of major organ functions (liver, bone, muscle, etc.) as well as metabolic pathways of nutrients such as glucose, protein, electrolytes and hormones. The information from these banks of tests can be helpful in the diagnosis, treatment and prevention of laminitis and founder.

Relationship of metabolic hormones and laminitis

Giving cortisone (cortisosteroid drugs) to horses at risk for laminitis is contraindicated (not advisable) as it causes the retention of fluids, which is the same laminitis-triggering effect as adrenal-released cortisol. Cortisol causes the body to retain sodium. Since water follows sodium, fluid migrates from the blood vessels into the tissues, producing further swelling and foot pain. If swelling and pain are not immediately relieved, laminitis may progress to pressure necrosis and founder.

The horse's system can give its own injection of cortisol from the adrenal glands located in front of the kidneys. With ingestion of an excessive amount of carbohydrates, or sugars, an increase in insulin and cortisol secretion occurs, which results in tissue edema by the same method that occurs when cortisone is administered.

Any stressful event, including endocrine and environmental changes, may also cause the release of cortisol by the adrenal glands, which results in edema due to the

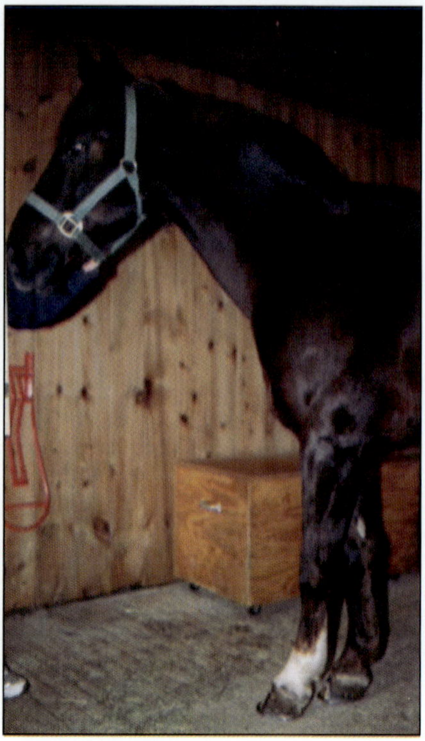

Figure 3-2. *Cresty neck of chronically foundered horse with Cushing's disease.* *© 2004 Doug Butler Enterprises, Inc. Used by permission.*

retention of sodium. When the swelling is in a closed vault such as the horse's foot, there is great pain and tissue damage. This is sometimes called "compartment syndrome" in human medicine.

Insulin resistance occurs when normal levels of insulin are not able to allow glucose to enter the cells. The pancreas responds to the resulting high blood glucose by secreting even more insulin. These horses are predisposed to laminitis presumably because the laminar tissue is starved for glucose. In addition, fat cells secrete hormones that hamper the action of

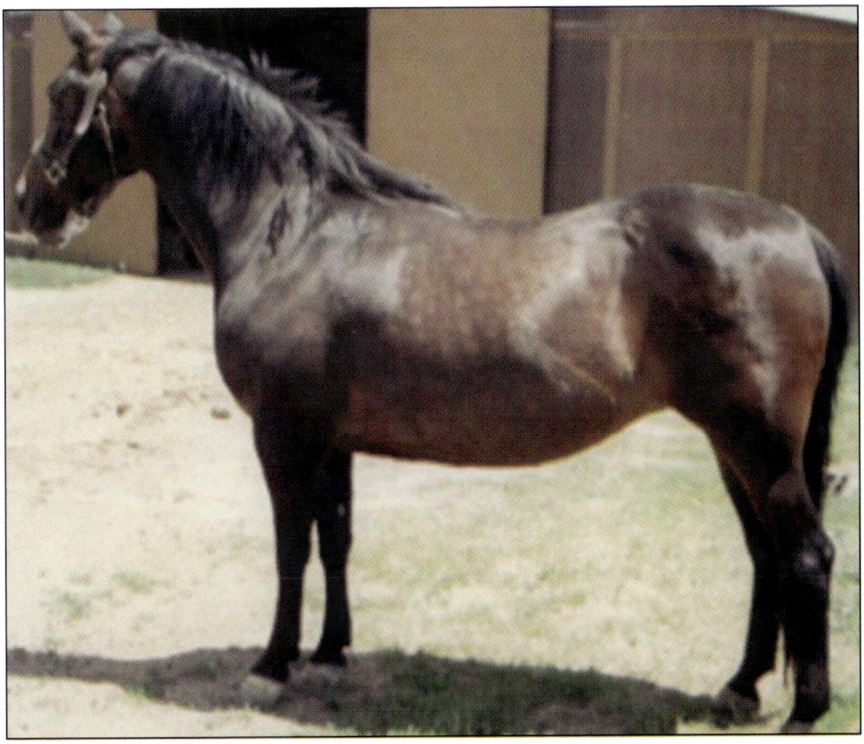

Figure 3-3. *Chronically foundered over-weight horse. © 2004 Doug Butler Enterprises, Inc. Used by permission.*

insulin (Treiber, Kronfeld, Hess, and Boston. *Amer. J. Vet. Research*. 66:2114-2121, 2005).

Dr. Pollitt's group in Australia found that twice as much force was required to separate laminar tissue with adequate glucose compared to that which didn't contain adequate glucose.

4

Relationships of Diet and the Equine Digestive Tract to Laminitis and Founder

The digestive system of the horse is in between a simple one, such as a human's, and a complex one, such as a cow's. Since horses have relatively small stomachs, they should be fed at regular times — at least twice a day — to prevent colic and oral vices such as wood chewing. Since horses are very anticipatory and strongly affected by habits, irregular feeding times may cause colic (gut ache) and can result in laminitis.

Horses are herbivores and are designed to graze grass for the majority of the 24-hour day. Their teeth, eye position, limb anatomy and digestive system contribute to this function. Horses are not designed to eat concentrated rations of high carbohydrate (sugar) content.

Pasture grass may be 70 percent moisture and only 30 percent dry matter. To get the amount of dry matter needed for body maintenance, a horse may eat three times as many pounds of grass as it would of hay (about 90 percent dry matter.)

Idle horses need between 1 to 2 percent of their body weight in dry feed per day. This amounts to about 10 to 20 pounds of hay per day for a 1,000-pound horse. For confined horses, this should be divided into two feedings at regular times to reduce the incidence of stable vices and colic.

Horses do not digest fiber as efficiently as ruminants, such as cows. In the horse, fermentation and the bacterial breakdown of fibrous feeds occurs in the large intestine after the feed passes through the small intestine. Horses depend upon the bacterial flora in the large intestine to ferment and digest fibrous feeds such as grass and hay.

Because intestinal bacteria need time to adapt from one type of feed to another, sudden changes in feed composition cause rapid fermentation and an increase in the acid content of the gut. Grasses with high sugar and fructan levels are desirable to increase meat production in ruminants, but often predispose idle horses to laminitis.

America's horse population is becoming older. Many geriatric animals are kept as pets and get very little exercise. The use of so-called "senior rations," high in molasses (sugar), starch (grains) and fat, often pose a risk to hypothyroid and cushingoid horses.

Feeding high energy feeds, combining supplements indiscriminately, allowing horses to graze clover pastures that may double in starch content in early spring, allowing equine access to the feed room, and other poor management practices may lead to laminitis.

Dietary or stress-related conditions

The progression of events leading to laminitis and founder resulting from dietary or stress-related conditions can be summarized as follows:

1) laminar tissues are acted upon by cortisol,

2) tissues swell,

3) blood vessels collapse,

4) lack of oxygen due to decreased blood flow causes tissue death,
5) death of cells and loss of structure causes release of enzymes,
6) enzymes cause the laminar basement membrane to come apart,
7) loss of integrity of laminae causes founder — rotating or sinking of the coffin bone.

Ingestion of a high sugar or fructan diet causes an increase in insulin and/or cortisol production by the body. (Stress causes a similar response). The presence of the sugar source causes an immediate and rapid fermentation and growth of Streptococcus bovis bacteria in the rear gut. Oxygen is depleted, creating an anaerobic condition and acidosis due to lactic acid production. The pH in the large intestine drops from 7 to 6.

The altered bacterial population of the gut produces increased levels of nitric oxide and fermentation gasses. This causes the smooth muscle of the gut and blood vessels to relax and dilate, producing gut stasis (stoppage of peristaltic movement). The bacteria also produce toxins that weaken the gut wall, enter into the blood and weaken the laminae. (Mungal, Kyaw-Tanner and Pollitt. *Vet. Microbiology*. 79:209-223, 2001).

The bacterial toxins and cortisol produced by the body cause the blood vessels in the closed vault of the foot to leak and the tissues to swell. The swelling tissues trapped between hoof and bone collapse the blood vessels, resulting in ischemia (lack of blood). Cells and tissues die as a result of the pressure necrosis and lack of circulation to the laminar tissues.

If present, arterial shunts (arteriovenous anastomoses-AVAs) in the foot may open to further divert blood from the laminar tissues (Pollitt and Molyneux. *Equine Vet. J.* 22(2): 79-87, 1990).

The dying cells release enzymes (matrix metalloproteinases-MMPs) from the laminae cell lysosomes, causing basement membranes between the sensitive and horny laminae to break down. The hoof/bone bond (laminar attachment) comes apart.

Pressure from the edema (swelling) pushes the hoof and bone apart and causes the hoof to deform. The coffin bone rotates and/or sinks in the hoof. The compression of the coronary band shuts off circulation at the toe, causing it to stop growing while the heel continues to grow.

Horses should be fed according to use and body condition

Horses should be fed according to work requirements and body condition. Most idle horses should be fed a limited amount of hay or pasture and do not need any grain in their daily ration. Monitor weight gain by sight, body condition scoring, equine scales, or a weight tape placed around the horse's girth.

When horses are allowed to eat too much, they enter into an anabolic state of metabolism and store fat. When they are burning more calories than they are fed, they are in a catabolic state. When the delicate balance is upset, the horse is at risk for laminitis.

When feeds are deficient in essential nutrients, horses cannot perform at optimum capacity. Hays that have been cured improperly or stored for a long period of time may be missing essential nutrients needed for normal metabolism and tissue growth.

Since modern horses are often overfed and do very little, if any, work, their situation could be compared to a person with a desk job eating like a professional athlete at a training table. The result will be fat storage and increased risk of metabolic diseases including laminitis.

All horses, ponies and donkeys are susceptible to laminitis. If more feed is available than is needed for maintenance, most equines will eat it, thus placing themselves at risk for laminitis. Ponies, in particular, are very susceptible to laminitis and founder because they weigh less and are 20 percent more efficient at digesting feed than are horses. (Breidbach, S. *Nutrition Reviews.* 30:259, 1959) Over-nutrition of idle horses causes greater than 50 percent of laminitis cases.

The 1998 National Animal Health Monitoring System Equine Study by the USDA–APHIS reported the causes of equine laminitis in the United States are due to:

46% Grazing lush pasture
7% Grain overload
3% Colic, diarrhea
2% Retained placenta
27% Known misc. (stress, poison, etc.)
15% Unknown

Fructans and laminitis

Fructans are compounds formed by grasses to store sugars formed by photosynthesis. The involvement of fructans in equine laminitis was first proposed by Dr. K. Hinkley of

England in 1997. Fructan composition can be as high as 40 percent of the dry matter of grass, according to K. Watts of Colorado. Ideally, they should be below 13 percent, yet regularly are in the 30 percent range in the early spring.

Researchers in Australia confirmed that high levels of fructans disrupt the balance of large intestine microflora, causing toxemia and activation of matrix metalloproteinase enzymes (MMPs) that degrade the basement membranes between the horny and sensitive laminae (Mungal, Kyaw-Tanner and Pollitt. *Vet. Microbiology*. 79:209-223, 2001).

Horses cannot absorb fructans in the small intestine. Excessive fructans passed to the hind gut lead to an imbalance of the microflora populations. Excessive consumption of grasses high in non-structural carbohydrates (NSCs) such as fructans, sugars and starches, whether in pastures or hays, create an acidic environment in the large intestine (lowering of the pH) when being acted upon by the bacteria. When the gut reaches the acidic pH of 6, the horse will usually become laminitic.

A horse's normal diet consists of grasses and hay containing typical levels of fructans, structural carbohydrates (SCs) and fiber. Fructans, SCs and fiber are digested in the large intestine by microbes. The beneficial end products are volatile fatty acids and other nutrients.

All forage is not the same

Plants and grasses can be grouped depending on one of two types of photosynthesis utilized. C3 photosynthesis is most efficient in cooler temperatures, therefore the C3 grasses are termed "cool season grasses." C4 photosynthesis occurs in "warm season grasses."

Cool season grasses (C3s) such as orchard, timothy, brome, crested wheat and blue grass have higher fructan content. Fescue and perennial rye grass are especially high. Even brown grasses in the winter can be high in fructans.

Warm-season grasses (C4s) such as Bermuda and Johnson grass are lower in fructans or non-structural carbohydrates (NSCs). Native prairie grasses have low levels of NSCs, but they are also low in production, since only one cutting of hay is harvested in a season

Warm-season grasses can accumulate fructans early in the growing season. Horses must be introduced slowly, a few hours at a time over the course of a week, to green pasture in the spring after eating hay during the winter months.

Growing grasses stressed by cold, drought or grazing will be high in fructans. Sunlight stimulates fructan production. Fructans are at their highest levels on warm days after cold days, late afternoon, sunny days, early spring, growing grass, during drought and at the base of freshly-grazed grass. They are lowest early in the morning.

Hay cut at a later stage has less nutrient value but is better for an idle horse. Processing the hay through a crusher cracks the stems, making the crop cure faster and be more digestible. Mixing lower quality hay with higher quality forage reduces the calorie content which is more suitable for an idle horse.

Hays made from grain crops such as oats, corn (maize), barley, wheat, rye and triticale should be avoided. Hay cuttings from the grain crops are high in carbohydrates and starch.

Fructan, starch and sugar content of grasses and hays can be analyzed at reasonable cost by a forage laboratory. Follow their instructions for collecting samples. Take several samples throughout the pasture season. Use the same laboratory all the way through the season to maintain consistency. Additional information and sources for grass analysis can be found at www.safergrass.org.

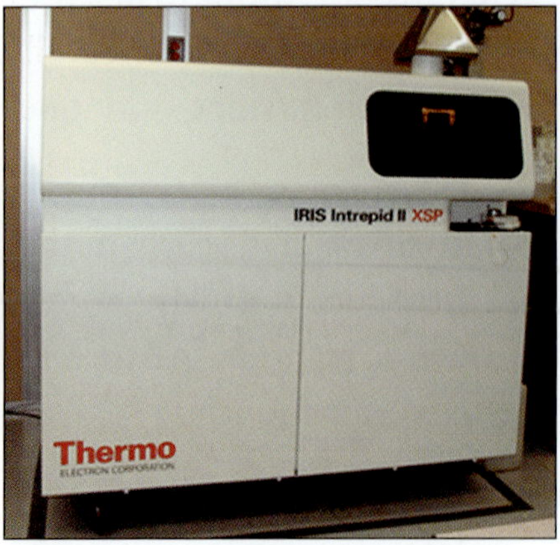

Figure 4-1. *ICP Spectrometer measures minerals and electrolytes. Photo provided by Life Data Labs Research Laboratory.*

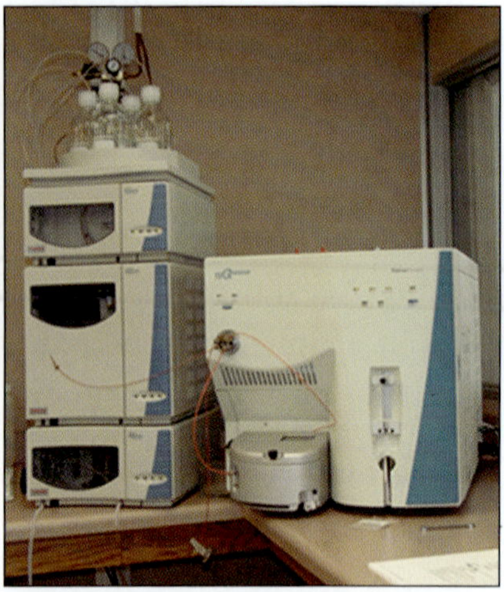

Figure 4-2. *Tandem HPLC / Mass Spectrometer measures lipids, sugars, proteins, amino acids and vitamins. Photo provided by Life Data Labs Research Laboratory.*

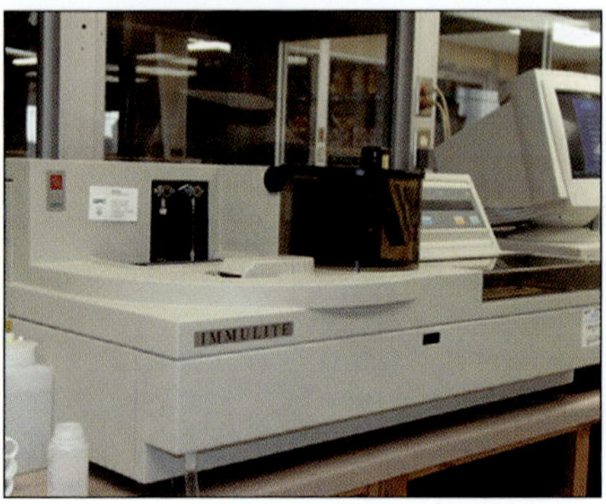

Figure 4-3. *Immunoassay analyzer measures hormones. Photo provided by Life Data Labs Research Laboratory.*

Feed supplementation helps repair damage from laminitis and founder

Many horses are being fed rations deficient in the nutrients necessary to maintain and rebuild their health. Many hays are deficient in essential nutrients, especially those put up after being rained on, grown on nutrient deficient soils or harvested at a late stage of maturity.

Horses that have had an attack of laminitis need a supplement that contains liver protectants and thyroid-positive nutrients. Amino acids play an important role in rebuilding a hoof damaged by laminitis and founder. Essential fatty acids are needed to build cell membranes and walls. Carotene and biotin are important hoof-building vitamins. Calcium, copper and zinc are important minerals for hoof strength. ***Note:*** For the individual nutrients furnished by proteins, essential fatty acids, vitamins and minerals to be most effective they must be both absorbable and in the proper ratio (balance).

Farrier's Formula® was created by veterinary nutrition specialist Dr. F. Gravlee using a mathematical modeling technique he began developing in 1979. He was formulating and testing prescription diets for growing, working and poor-footed horses. Blood analysis profiles were obtained and reviewed every six months on more than one hundred horses over a period of 10 years. Since Farrier's Formula's® introduction in 1982, four hundred more horses have been added to the profile database verifying the efficacy of the product.

The unique formula combines the hoof-building nutrients that are necessary to rebuild a strong hoof after tissue damage occurs during laminitis. The hoof needs to be strong to protect the fragile coffin bone within the foot, much like the skull protects the brain. This is why barefoot is not a good idea for horses that are ridden and worked under adverse conditions, especially those that have genetically weak or damaged hooves.

5

Diagnosis, Prevention and Prognosis of Laminitis

With laminitis, several conditions may appear all at once. It is important to recognize laminitis as an emergency, treat the symptoms immediately and work to prevent future occurrences.

Early in the course of the laminitis, edema is the main problem. To reduce swelling and prevent further swelling of the sensitive foot tissues, encourage the horse to lie down in a deep bed of shavings. Do not give the horse any Bute.

To reduce inflammation and prevent further damage to the hoof coriums (tissues that grow the hoof capsule, the wall, sole and frog) determine the condition that created the laminitis component and remove or neutralize it.

After the tissues have been damaged and the horse has foundered, it is important to position and support the damaged structures so the body can repair them. This repair process is often slower than we would like.

And finally, the destroyed tissue must be rebuilt by feeding a diet proven to improve dermal tissue.

Classifying laminitis and founder based on diagnostic signs

To allow effective diagnosis and treatment, laminitis must be recognized in its different stages. Laminitis may result from insults to the laminae from various sources, including infectious disease. Upon initial examination, the classification must be determined in order to choose proper management and treatment.

Mild laminitis

- Swelling in the lower legs.
- Coronet (top of the hoof) is warmer than the rest of the body.
- Digital pulse is slightly increased in rate and amplitude (throbbing).
- Elevated blood levels of ACTH, plasma cortisol, insulin and triglycerides.
- Soles may be painful when compressed with hoof testers.
- Gait will be off and the horse may refuse jumps; behavior will favor the feet.

Acute laminitis

- Horses affected in the front feet will rock back on their hind feet pushing their front feet forward and head up in an effort to relieve pressure from the swelling feet. Those affected in the hind feet will stand over the front legs with the head down. Those affected in one foot will rest or hold up that leg, and those affected in all four feet will act like they are glued to the ground.
- The soles will be painful when compressed with hoof testers.
- The digital pulse is increased in rate and amplitude (throbbing).

- There are elevated blood levels of ACTH, plasma cortisol, insulin and triglycerides.
- Radiographs may reveal a slight rotation and/or sinking of the coffin bone.

Mild chronic founder

- The white line (yellow) will be wider than its normal width of 1/8th inch.
- The hoof wall may be distorted with a dished dorsal wall and growth rings wider apart at the heels.
- Radiographs will reveal rotation and/or sinking of the coffin bone, but the tip of the coffin bone is sharp and the dorsal surface is not rough.
- These horses are often overweight. Hard, cresty neck and fat deposits over the loin and tail head may indicate equine metabolic syndrome.
- Puffiness over the eyes often occurs with hypothyroidism.
- Impaired thyroid function occurs as a hormone response to chronic high grain feeding (increased blood cortisol level is a contributing factor.)
- Impaired thyroid function from long term "Bute" therapy.
- Long hair that won't shed (hirsutism) with increased drinking and urinating caused by a pituitary tumor (Cushing's disease).
- Painful teeth and gums (periodontal disease) caused by Cushing's disease.

Severe chronic founder

- Radiographs will reveal significant founder distance (distance from top of hoof wall to top of extensor process of the coffin bone) indicating sinking of the coffin bone. A depression can be felt by running your finger down the front of the pastern to the coronary band. (See Figure 5-2 on page 53.)
- Radiographs will reveal P3 bone demineralization, sinking and possible penetration of the sole. The bone tip will not be sharp and may be absent. The dorsal surface may be rough.
- The sole will be flattened or dropped (convex). Lameness will persist.
- The hoof wall will be distorted with a dished dorsal wall and with growth rings wider apart at the heel, which usually indicates contraction of deep flexor muscles are reducing growth of toe and increasing growth of heel.
- Knuckling over and contraction of the superficial flexor muscles may indicate pain in the coffin bone caused by osteomyelitis (bone infection).

Preventing laminitis

Laminitis and founder are two of the most severe foot lamenesses that afflict horses. If laminitis is not recognized and treated as an emergency, most laminitis cases will turn into founder cases. Prevention of laminitis is more successful than treatment!

Here are seven ways to help prevent laminitis.

1) **Feed a consistent quality and quantity of feeds.** Give at least two feedings per day. Mismanagement due to overfeeding idle horses causes 70 to 80 percent of laminitis cases.

   Horses have strong instinctive appetites. This characteristic serves them well in the wild. They spend the majority of a 24-hour day grazing low-calorie forages. They move with a herd and get adequate exercise to burn up the calories in their feed.

   When domesticated, a horse's dominant grazing behavior is altered. If confined, they often develop vices with their mouths such as wood chewing and cribbing. If left on a lush pasture loaded with nutrients and calories, they may literally eat themselves to death. Free-choice grazing of sparse vegetation in the wild sustains them, while free-choice grazing in a fertilized and growing pasture can kill them.

   It's much easier to kill a horse with kindness in the form of too much feed than it is to hurt it by feeding it too little. Neither of these alternatives is good. To do what is best for the horse, you must understand its physiology.

   The horse has a relatively small stomach (about 10 percent of its digestive tract) that is designed to hold small amounts eaten frequently. For this reason it is a good practice to feed horses at least twice a day when they are confined to avoid colic (stomach ache).

   Horses live in a dominance hierarchy. It's best to feed each horse individually because a dominant animal will get too much feed, while a less-dominant one may get too little. If feeding individually is not possible or practical, place the feed in spaced-out individual piles, with as many piles as there are horses.

Each idle horse needs only about 1-1/2 percent of its body weight in quality hay per day. This means a 1,000-pound horse should get about 15 pounds of hay per day. If this is divided into two feedings, the horse should get about 7-1/2 pounds each morning and each evening. Most string-tied bales weigh about 60 pounds. Since 15 goes into 60 four times, in this example, a bale should last four days. In other words, this horse should be fed 1/8th of a bale at each feeding. Variance in hay quality may necessitate adjusting the amount fed depending upon whether the horse gains or loses weight.

2) **Make provision for idle horses to exercise.**

3) **Check condition and monitor weight** with a scale or weight tape.

   Confine overweight horses to a dry lot with limited feed intake and no access to growing pasture. Adipose tissue can act as an endocrine organ to synthesize and secrete the inflammatory cytokine TN∝. Excess adipose tissue is a major contributor to the development of insulin resistance (Vick and Fitzgerald. Univ. of Kentucky. 15(2-Apr):5, 2006).

4) **Limit fructan intake** by limiting grazing on sunny days after cool nights. Analyze pasture and hay grasses to determine levels of starch and fructans. Ideally, fructan levels should be below 13 percent in grass hay. Directions for testing hays can be obtained at www.safergrass.org.

5. **Eliminate molasses and grains** from the diet of at-risk horses. Idle horses rarely need grain. Grain is most useful to

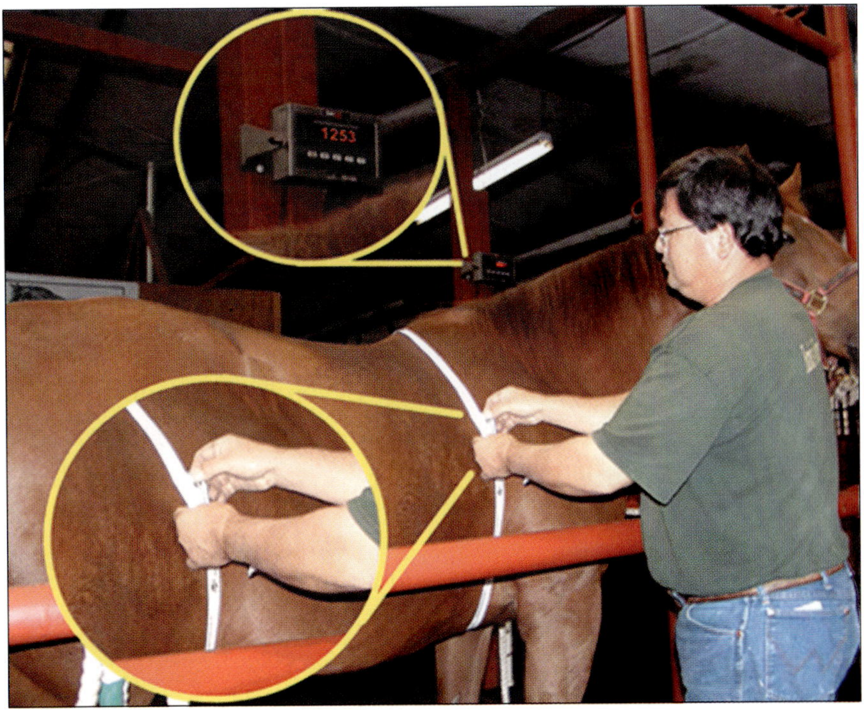

Figure 5-1. *The most accurate procedure for measuring weight is the electronic scale; however, the weight tape is the most commonly-used method. Top circle shows enlarged detail of digital readout mounted on post behind the horse; lower circle shows enlarged detail of using a weight tape. Photo provided by Life Data Labs Equine Nutrition Research Farm.*

catch horses and to put weight on thin horses. Concentrated feeds high in sugar and starches are especially dangerous to older horses with Cushing's disease.

6. **Introduce any feed changes gradually** over the course of a week.

7. **Avoid toxins,** such as found in black walnut shavings, and situations perceived as stressful by the horse, when possible.

Prognostic indicators of laminitis

The prognosis of a laminitic horse is influenced by the degree (grade) of lameness, radiographic or other diagnostic tests, and physical examination. Prognosis improves with early and proper intervention.

Lameness classifications

Lameness is defined and graded by number. The American Association of Equine Practitioners adopted the following classification in 1984 (*Guide for Veterinary Service and Judging of Equestrian Events–AAEP Newsletter.* 3:24, June, 1984).

Definition: Lameness is a deviation from normal gait or posture due to pain or mechanical dysfunction.

Grade Classifications

Grade 1: Difficult to observe; not consistently apparent regardless of circumstances (i.e. weight-carrying, circling, inclines, hard surface, etc.).

Grade 2: Difficult to observe at a walk or in trotting a straight line; consistently apparent under certain circumstances (i.e. weight-carrying, circling, inclines, hard surface, etc.).

Grade 3: Consistently observable at a trot under all circumstances.

Grade 4: Obvious lameness: marked nodding, hitching or shortened stride.

Grade 5: Minimal weight-bearing in motion and/or at rest; inability to move (appears glued to the ground).

Radiographic indicators

The radiographic distance from the top of the extensor process of the coffin bone to the top of the coronary band was described by Burney Chapman as an important prognostic measurement. This can be a significantly better prognostic indicator to predict a horse's chance of recovery than is bone rotation or sole perforation. As the founder distance increases, the chance the horse has for complete recovery decreases.

Physical examination indicators

A useful technique to determine the relative founder distance without a radiograph is to run your finger down the front of the pastern to the hoof. If it slips over the coronary band easily, the founder distance is low or insignificant. If your finger drops in a depression at the toe, the founder distance is greater and the chances for complete recovery are lower. If there are also depressions on the sides of the coronary band, the horse is probably a sinker with the lowest chance of recovery.

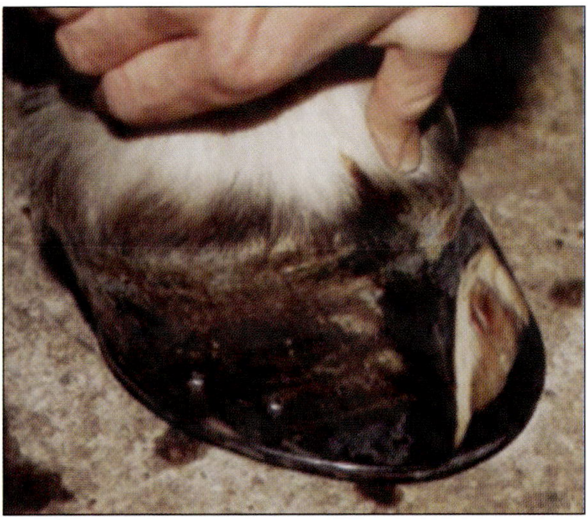

Figure 5-2. *A sinker can be identified by pushing your thumb in at the coronary band. This indicates the coffin bone has sunk in the hoof. Normally, the thumb will slide off. Photo © 2004 Doug Butler Enterprises, Inc. Used by permission.*

6

Clinical or Medical Treatment and Management of Laminitis and Founder

Laminitis and founder is a complicated systemic disease that severely affects a horse's feet. Dr. D. Jolly (*Amer. Farriers J.* July/Aug, 1986) said, "Any farrier or veterinarian who decides to tackle founder alone, without the cooperation of the other, does not have the best interest of the animal nor of the owner in mind."

Dr. C. Colles of England (*Equine Vet. J.* 23:4, 1991) said: "There seems to be little doubt that a heart bar shoe, correctly fitted by a skilled farrier, is a great help in treating founder … However, shoeing cannot cure a systemic disease … Veterinarians seem to be opting out of treating laminitis/founder and delegating or abrogating their responsibilities to the farrier. Many farriers, perhaps unwisely, are rising to the challenge … A joint approach by professionals with mutually synergistic talents must give the horse its best chance of recovery."

Veterinarians and farriers must work together for the best chance of recovery

Farriers and veterinarians who work together must be committed to solving the horse's problem and be able to overlook differences caused by any previous misunderstandings. The horse owner pays for the knowledge and work necessary to restore a horse to health and, therefore, has the right to insist on harmony and performance.

When interviewing farriers and vets, ask each of them if they have someone they routinely work with on laminitis/founder cases. If they cannot name someone they recommend, keep searching. You are looking for a team that can work together with you to solve a very complex and potentially deadly problem. Farriers may understand the mechanical aspects of the problem, but not the medical aspects. Veterinarians may understand the medical aspects, but not the mechanical.

A combination of medical and mechanical treatments is necessary to solve a horse's problem when it is foundered. The cause must be determined and the swelling, pain and systemic condition(s) treated. The bone column must be supported while the horse grows a new hoof.

Founder can be compared to a human smashing his or her fingernail. The nail/bone bond is destroyed and a person needs to grow a new nail to protect the end of the finger. Unlike the human, the horse stands and walks on its fingernail, complicating recovery. The temporary transfer of weight to the frog provides support to the bone column while the injured toe wall (fingernail) grows back.

Recommended clinical management and treatments

The object of medical treatments is to reduce swelling and prevent loss of blood vessel integrity.

• **Treat acute cases as an emergency.**

• **Determine and treat the cause** to stop the progressive damage, and to help prevent future occurrences.

• **Evacuate the bowel** with a purgative such as mineral oil with an added anti-microbial when the cause is digestive tract in origin. (This also blocks absorption and production of toxins.)

• **Soak feet in ice cold water** in a creek bed or boots with ice cream salt to cool the feet for several days. The cold constricts the over-dilated laminar blood vessels, thereby retarding the formation of edema and pressure within the hoof vault. It also decreases the oxygen requirement by decreasing the metabolic rate — prolonging the life of the tissues.

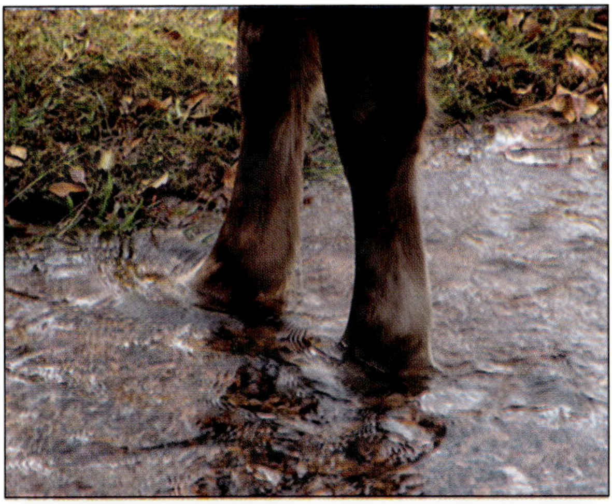

Figure 6-1. *(top) Standing a horse in cold running water has been the accepted standard laminitis treatment for hundreds of years.*

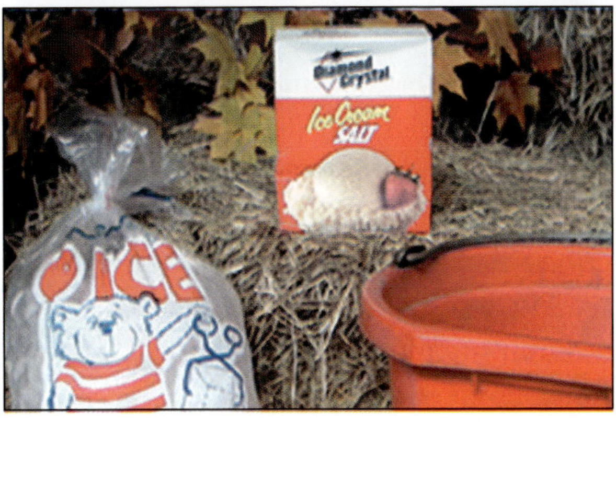

Figure 6-2. *(bottom) Since the advent of refrigeration and ice-making, we have been able to bring "cold treatment" to the horse. Photos provided by Life Data Labs Equine Nutrition Research Farm.*

• **Slowly move the horse's head** from side to side to gently shift weight from one foot to the other. This helps prevent circulatory stagnation.

• **Inject Ergonovine or oxytocin** (powerful blood vessel constrictors) as indicated for three or four days. The increased vessel muscle tone helps prevent blood from leaking from the vessels and helps prevent their collapse. This drug is not to be used on pregnant or lactating mares, nor when fescue toxicity is suspected.

• **Inject Dipyrone** (Metamizole) (banned from human medicine and food animals), an anti-inflammatory that doesn't sedate, usually twice a day in the muscle. Aspirin given orally can be substituted as a short-term treatment. Anti-histamines also help reduce temperature and inflammation. "Bute" (phenylbutazone) is not recommended because it has a pain-killing effect which will discourage the horse from lying down, and the horse will lose the benefit of keeping its feet at the same level as its heart.

• **Brush DMSO** on the entire foot from the fetlock down, including the skin and hair below the fetlock, the hoof wall, the sole and the frog. It is rapidly absorbed and reduces swelling.

• **Use Robaxin-V** (Methocarbamol) to relax skeletal muscles (including the superficial and deep flexors) enabling the horse to unlock its legs, thus encouraging the horse to lie down. Administer in the vein initially, followed by intramuscular injections each 8 hours as indicated. Continue Robaxin as necessary to allow the flexor muscles to relax. We do not recommend tenotomy (cutting the tendon). Laminitis is not a disease of the deep flexor tendon!

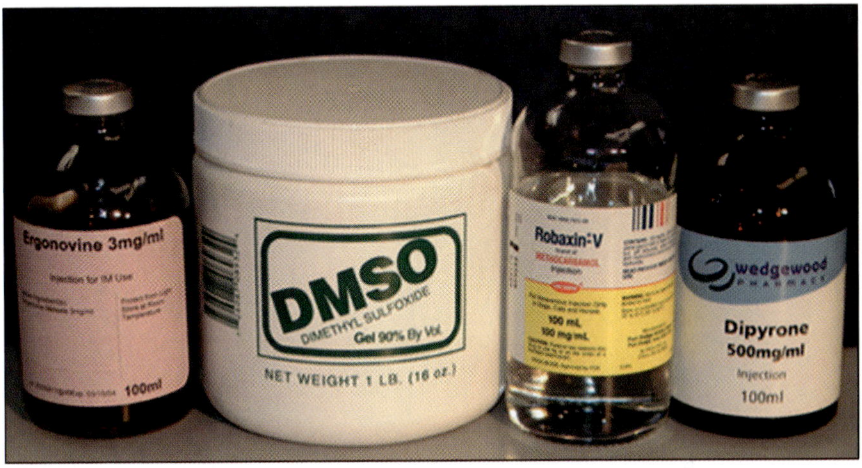

Figure 6-3. *Four drugs successfully used in the treatment of laminitis are (from left): Ergonovine, DMSO, Robaxin-V and Dipyrone. Photo provided by Life Data Labs Research Laboratory.*

• **Resection (remove) a section of the dorsal hoof wall** to relieve swelling, release pressure from the coronary band and drain abscesses. Grooving the hoof wall and sole, first described by the French, was recommended by Dr. E. Frank in *Veterinary Surgery* as far back as 1939. It was revived by B. Chapman and G. Platt in the late 1960s.

• **Prescribe heart bar shoes.** These should be reset once a month to reestablish hoof angle and uniform frog contact.

• **Encourage the horse to lie down** in a deep bed of shavings (18 inches). Forced walking is contraindicated (not advisable).

• **Offer free choice water,** limit grass hay consumption, and do not feed grain.

• **Prescribe Farrier's Formula®** to aid the body in healing diseased tissue.

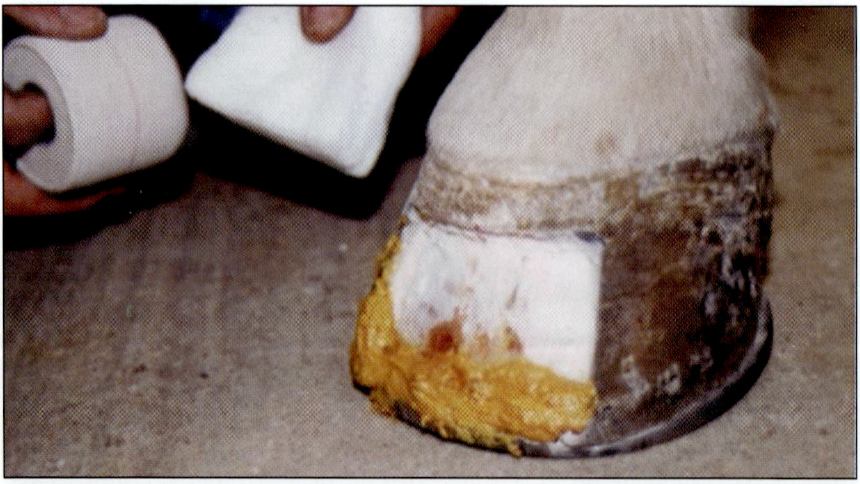

Figure 6-4. *Extensive resection of dorsal hoof wall to drain abscesses and allow normal hoof growth of wall. © 2004 Doug Butler Enterprises, Inc. Used by permission.*

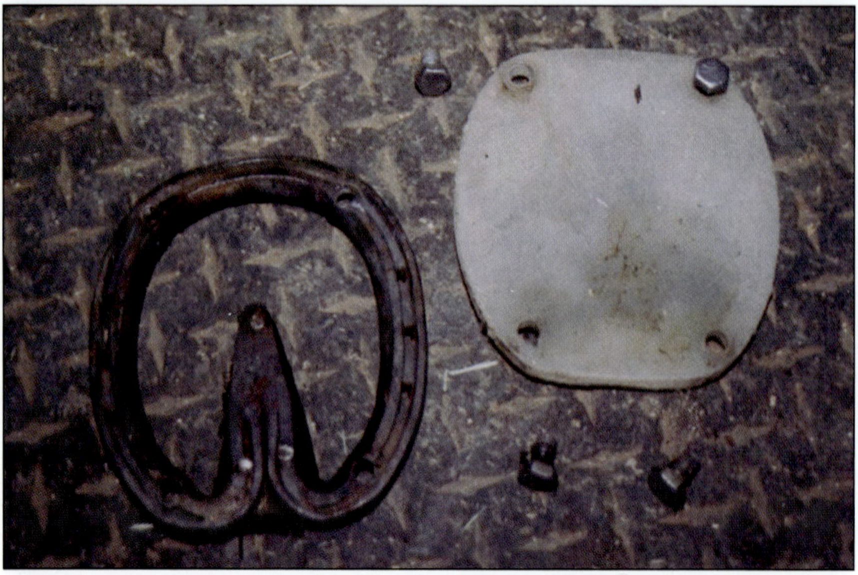

Figure 6-5. *Heart bar shoes help reestablish hoof angle and uniform frog contact. A hospital plate (on right) protects an exposed coffin bone and holds in medication. © 2004 Doug Butler Enterprises, Inc. Used by permission.*

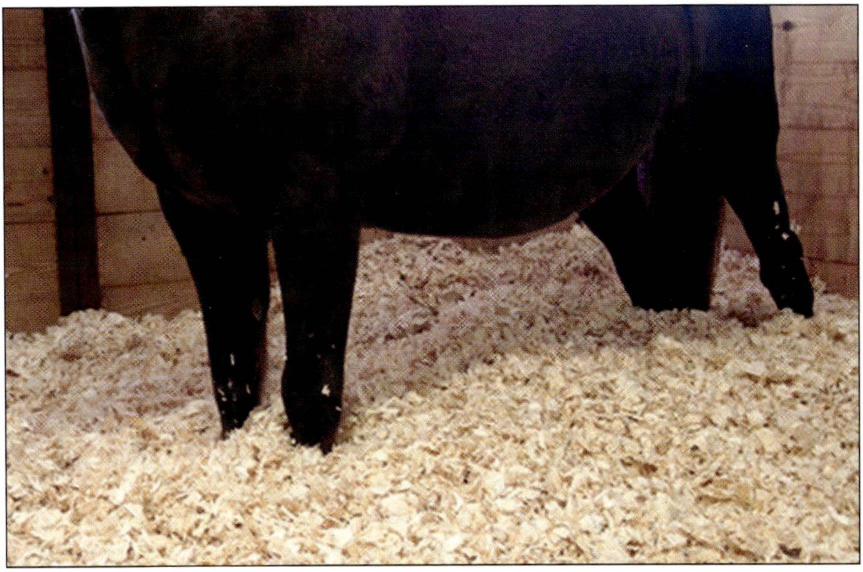

Figure 6-6. *The horse should be encouraged to lie down in a deep bed of shavings (18 inches minimum). Photo provided by Life Data Labs Equine Nutrition Research Farm.*

Other drugs that can be used when indicated include:

Dextran — Increases osmotic pressure in the blood plasma and encourages fluid to move from the edematous tissue and return to circulation.

Lasix — Diuretic that helps pull fluid out of the tissues, which reduces tissue edema.

Eq Stim — Boosts system immunity and may help prevent osteomyelitis.

Baytril, Ampicillin and/or Gentamycin — Antibiotics, indicated if infection is present.

Prognosis

When attention and detail is given to treatment for laminitis and founder, all but the most seriously affected will improve dramatically, although some cases will take longer than others. Mechanical support with therapeutic shoes may be required for several months or, rarely, years.

7

Understanding the Anatomy of the Horse's Foot Assists in Treating Laminitis and Founder

Horses have a stay apparatus in their limbs which allows them to graze standing for long periods of time and rest standing up. The arrangement of tendons and ligaments allows the horse, with very little muscular effort, to lock its limb joints and rest the large muscle groups that support its weight.

In the front limb, the leg is locked by the arrangement of opposing tendons and ligaments, the eccentric elbow joint and a slight muscle tonus on the triceps muscle. In the hind leg, the leg is locked by the arrangement of opposing tendons and ligaments, the position of the medial patellar ligament over the trochlea of the femur and a slight muscle tonus on the tensor fasciae latae muscle on the patella. In addition, the hind leg has a reciprocal apparatus that assures that the stifle, hock and fetlock joints all flex together.

When a horse experiences the severe foot pain of laminitis, the limb muscles tense up and lock the limbs in the standing position. It becomes very difficult for an afflicted horse to lie down and take the weight off its feet. Robaxin is helpful in this situation. In addition, since horses are preyed-upon animals, they instinctively resist lying down as they fear they will be vulnerable to attack while incapacitated.

Deep bedding (18 inches of shavings is recommended) and using no pain-killing drugs encourage a laminitic horse to lie down. The object is to get the weight off of the feet and get them on the same level as or above the heart. Dr. E. Frank, in *Veterinary Surgery*, recommended casting a horse with laminitis to keep the weight off the feet.

The anatomy of the foot must be understood to effectively treat laminitis

The coriums or sensitive structures of the foot produce the various parts of the hoof. The outer layers of the hoof wall are produced at the coronary band and grow downward. The upper portion of inner layer of the hoof wall, called the insensitive laminae, is produced exclusively from the coronary corium but about 20 to 30 percent of the lower portion of the hoof wall is produced by the sensitive laminae.

The sensitive laminae on the distal phalanx or coffin bone interlock with the insensitive lamina on the inner hoof wall. This arrangement allows the hoof to grow downward but still remain attached to the bone. A healthy attachment is so strong that all weight-bearing can be removed from the sole and frog, and the bone column remains suspended from the hoof wall by the laminae. Thus, we see the wall is anatomically designed to carry the major portion of a horse's weight.

The hoof wall is designed to bear weight through a Velcro-like hoof-bone bond formed by the laminae. There are 500 to 600 primary laminae and 100 to 200 secondary laminae on each primary lamina in a healthy horse foot. Each lamina looks like a feather when cross-sectioned and viewed under the microscope.

This design of the laminar attachment increases the surface area of the hoof-bone bond so that less weight is distributed over each part of its surface. Dr. H. Möller, a German veterinarian quoted by G. Fleming in *The Veterinarian* in the 1870s, measured and calculated the laminar area at 8 square feet per foot in a mature light horse. This amounts to about 4 ounces per square inch of attachment, instead of the several hundred pounds per square inch that would be stressing the bone if weight were transferred directly from a simple union of bone to hoof.

The coffin or distal phalanx bone is very fragile due to its porosity caused by the blood vessels and nerves that permeate it. Its lightness on the end of a long leg bone column helps prevent fatigue in the running horse. The hoof is designed to contain and protect the bone within it from injury. Hence, the name coffin bone.

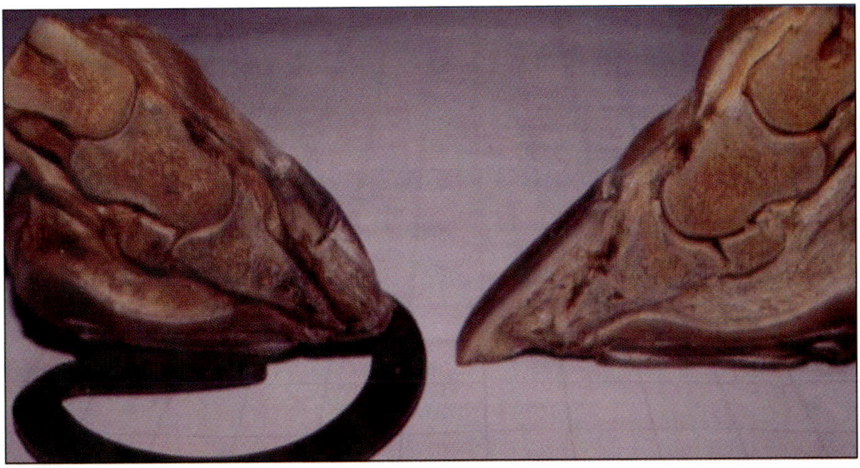

Figure 7-1. *Cross-section of freeze-dried specimen showing trimming and fit of heart bar (no weight on toe) and extent of resection on a severe sinker. (Untrimmed right; trimmed and shod left) Photo © 2004 Doug Butler Enterprises, Inc. Used by permission.*

The laminar hoof-bone attachment has two sources of blood supply

The sensitive laminae have a rich blood supply. C. Richardson of England, in his *Practical Farriery* published in 1950, stated that more blood goes through the horse's foot each minute than goes through its brain. Blood is needed to repair damaged tissues, provide for normal growth and create a hydraulic cushion between the two hard substances: hoof and bone.

Blood vessels are located between the bone and hoof. When the laminar attachment is weak, as in some poor-footed Thoroughbreds and Warm Bloods, the hoof-bone bond comes apart, tearing the blood vessels, allowing the tip of the bone to sink and constrict the circumflex artery.

When the laminar attachment is destroyed as in laminitis and founder, lack of blood supply and vessel leaking causes swelling and constriction of blood vessels producing tissue death called necrosis. Necrotic tissue turns into abscesses that produce heat, swelling and pain.

Normally, the majority of the blood supply to the laminae comes from the digital arteries into the terminal arch and through the porous coffin bone. The blood supply to the laminae also comes up from the circumflex artery and to a lesser extent down from the coronary band.

The blood supply to the sole comes from the circumflex artery. Foundered horses usually have dry blood or serum-stained soles due to internal bruising of and a lack of blood supply to the sole. There are no blood vessels coming through the bottom of the distal phalanx or coffin bone. The blood vessels come through the dorsal surface of the bone and anastomose (join) with the circumflex artery around the outside edge of the bone.

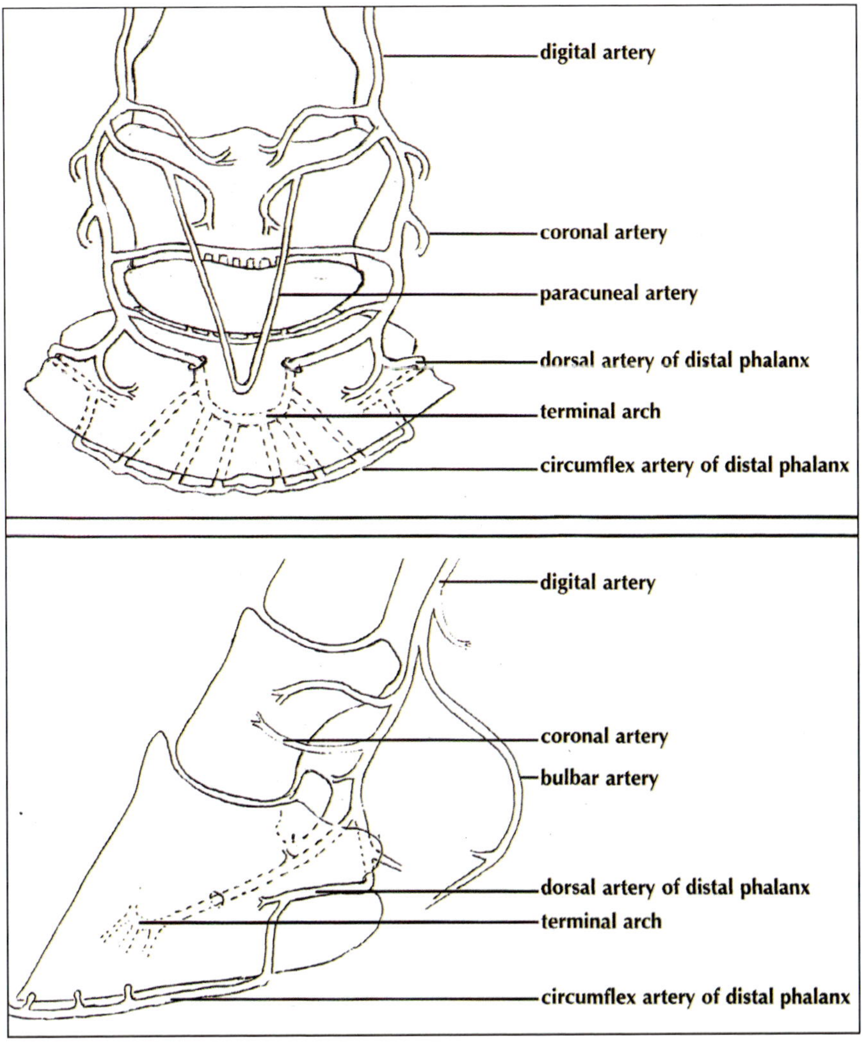

Figures 7-2, 7-3. *The arteries of a horse's foot. Illustration © 2004 Doug Butler Enterprises, Inc. Used by permission.*

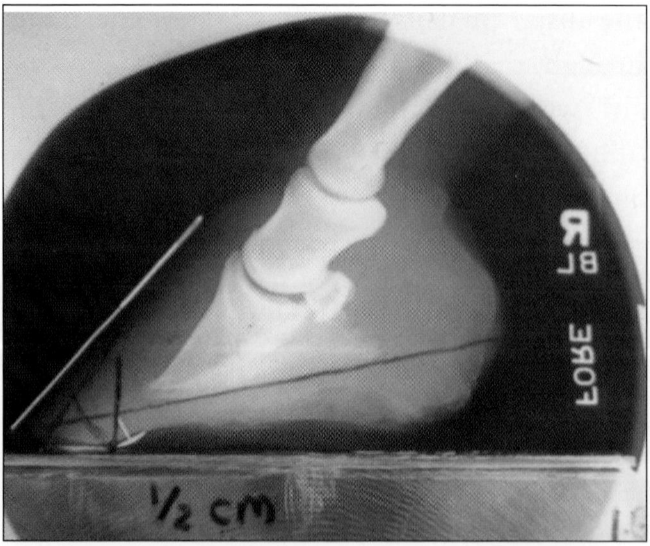

Figure 7-4. *A radiograph shows the position of the coffin bone and remodeling. Photo © 2004 Doug Butler Enterprises, Inc. Used by permission.*

Dr. C. Pollitt of Australia (*Equine Foot Studies* video, 1992) has demonstrated an alternative circulation coming from the dorsal artery at the rear of the coffin bone that is activated when weight bearing is shifted from the wall to the frog. The support of the bone supplied by the frog allows the circumflex artery at the toe to fill and repair the sensitive laminae and sole.

Reduced blood supply causes bone remodeling and pain

The condition of the tip of the coffin or distal phalanx bone as viewed on a radiograph is a good indicator of the potential success of any founder treatment.

A normal tip of the distal phalanx forms a sharp point when viewed laterally. The tip of the distal phalanx bone of a foundered horse will remodel and even be absorbed over an extended period of time. Bone remodeling indicates there is less chance of a pain-free recovery.

Lack of blood supply to an area (called ischemia) is painful. Apparently the process of remodeling can only be stopped or slowed and not reversed. Rarely will horses afflicted with bone changes become totally pain free.

Once the bone becomes infected (called osteomyelitis), the horse can rarely be saved since a lack of blood supply prevents antibiotics from reaching the infection.

The blood vessels passing through the bone to the laminae from the terminal arch of the digital arteries are stretched and destroyed by the swelling and downward movement of the bone when a horse founders. The blood supply is cut off due to the rotation (at toe) or sinking (all around) of the distal phalanx. Circulation cannot be reestablished until the weight borne on the toe constricting the circumflex artery is transferred to the rear of the foot.

8

Shoeing or Mechanical Treatment and Management of Laminitis and Founder

Many mechanical treatment options have been used successfully to treat laminitis and founder problems. However, few have proven to work with any degree of consistency. Many times, perhaps as much as 80 percent of the time, the horse had a strong enough constitution and hoof that it would have gotten better in spite of the "treatment." Ten percent may die no matter what you do, but 10 percent will recover only with expert medical and mechanical help and competent nursing.

Shoeing neglected foundered horses (said to be chronically foundered) is not an accurate test of any mechanical treatment method, as most of these animals will usually improve with only trimming. Shoes other than the heart bar shoe will work occasionally, but not with any degree of consistency. Some horses can tolerate bad farriery better than others.

Burney Chapman and Dr. George Platt, reporting their experience since 1968 on hundreds of horses to the American Association of Equine Practitioners Convention in 1984, indicated that none of the following mechanical treatments worked with any degree of consistency (*AAEP Proceedings* 30: 99-109, 1984). Yet, many are still advocated by modern farrier and veterinarian practitioners.

Chapman and Platt reported that none of the mechanical treatments listed below was as consistently effective for mechanically treating founder as a precisely fitted heart bar shoe. This has been our experience as well.

1) Egg bar shoe
2) Reverse shoe
3) Reverse wedge pad
4) Hoof cast
5) Shoe with bar across shoe center
6) Pad with packing against sole
7) Shoe that raises the heel

Mechanical treatments: Trimming

Trimming forms the foundation of a therapeutic shoeing job.

The distorted hoof wall should be rasped until its outer surface is parallel to the dorsal surface of the distal phalanx bone. The axis of the phalanx bones should be in balance or in line when viewed from the side. Dr. O. Balch and others have determined that the least amount of stress is placed upon the leg structures when the axes of the phalanges are aligned (Balch, Ratzlaff, Hyde and White. *AAEP Proceedings*, 37:687-705, 1991). Bone position can be accurately determined from lateral radiographs.

The distribution of weight must be as uniform as possible over the ground surface area of the frog. The frog must be trimmed until it is soft. Large frogs are trimmed level with the ground surface or the hoof wall; small frogs need a build-up.

Frog build-ups are made by building up the space between the bar and frog with leather or plastic shims riveted to the heart bar. Injector-mixed or hand-mixed frog support composite can also be used under the bar to fill the space between the frog and shoe. The horse should stand on the shoe before the mixed materials set up to allow excess to ooze out the back.

Sole pressure (sometimes called sole support) is contraindicated (not advisable). Standing a horse in sand does not help since the sensitive sole is very vascular. Pressure applied over the entire sole can further limit circulation and cause complications. Applying sole pressure causes the horse to stand on what hurts. At first it may seem to offer pain relief, just as head pressing is resorted to when horses or people have head pain due to swelling inside the skull, but eventually the horse will be worse off after more tissue is destroyed due to a compromised blood supply.

Thinning the sole allows it to flex and relieve swelling pressure. Care must be exercised so as not to perforate the sole as the result will be exuberant granulation tissue. A hospital plate between the shoe and ground is required when the sole is perforated or painful.

Dorsal wall resections should be done after the shoes are applied. Resections relieve fluid pressure under the laminar wedge and help restore the blood supply to the front of the coronary band in addition to relieving pressure from abscesses and seromas.

Mechanical treatment: Shoeing with a heart bar shoe

The most consistently effective mechanical treatment to supplement medical treatment is the heart bar shoe re-introduced in our generation by the late AFA certified journeyman farrier Burney Chapman of Texas. This has been verified in clinical practice as well as articles in scientific journals. Good farriery makes all the difference.

An understanding of the vascular anatomy of the foot is necessary to successfully apply the heart bar shoe to a foundered foot. The farrier applying it must be qualified to do this work, meaning he or she has had successful experiences with this kind of shoeing.

The heart bar shoe, correctly fitted to the foot, transfers a portion of the horse's weight from the wall to the frog. The corium of the frog has a comparatively small blood supply, compared to the corium of the laminae and the corium of the sole.

The heart bar shoe supports the distal phalanx bone, like an arch support in a human shoe, allowing blood to enter and flow through the previously constricted circumflex artery by the alternate route via the dorsal artery at the rear of the distal phalanx.

The nails used should be of a light slim blade design (such as MX50 or 5 Slim or smaller) and placed in the rear of the hoof behind the point of the heart bar. No nails should be placed in the toe area.

Fitting of the heart bar shoe must be precise

The pressure placed against the frog by the heart bar is determined by feel. Some experience is required to get it right. The shoe should be squeezed down against the frog using

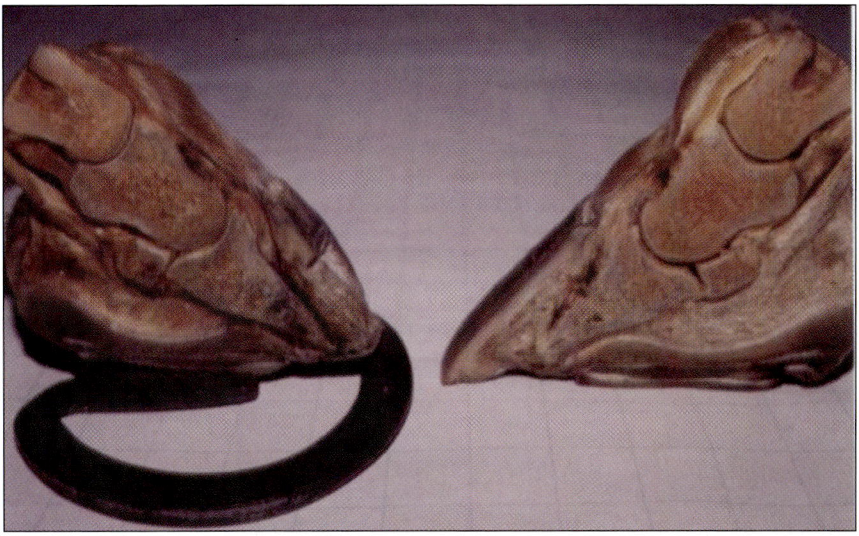

Figure 8-1. *Cross-section of foot bones that have been cut in half to show the fit of a heart bar and extent of resection (no weight on toe) on a severe sinker compared to its unshod cross section. Photo © 2004 Doug Butler Enterprises, Inc. Used by permission.*

thumb pressure. The force required to slightly compress the frog and rest the shoe solidly on the wall is about right for most horses. Two nails are driven, the foot is put down, and the horse is allowed to bear weight on it.

The horse is observed for signs of comfort or discomfort. Resting an alternate foot or expressing a big sigh of relief as the horse loads the foot are good signs. The lower jaw loosens up and the horse often moves its tongue when it's relaxed. In comparison, starting to load the foot and then backing off and resting it, as well as tension around the mouth, are bad signs. The shoe must be removed and the bar readjusted until it is right. An accurate reading of the horse's condition can only be obtained when no painkillers are used while shoeing the horse.

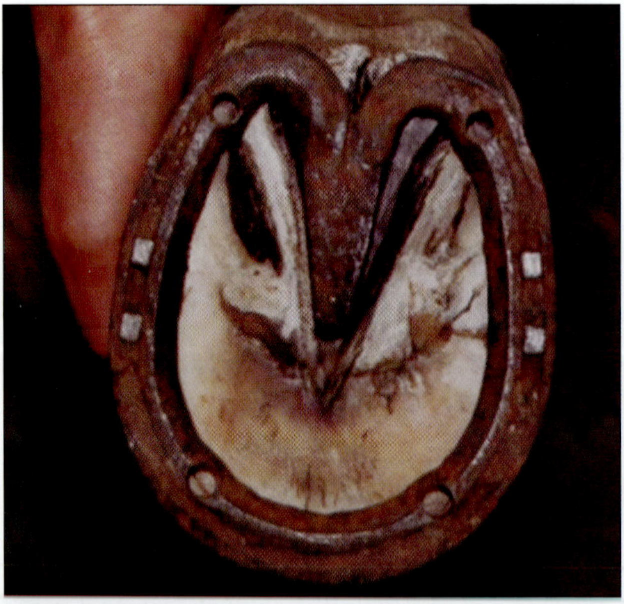

Figure 8-2. *Heart bar shoe drilled and tapped for hospital plate showing correct fit around frog. Note the discoloration of sole in front of frog. © 2004 Doug Butler Enterprises, Inc. Used by permission.*

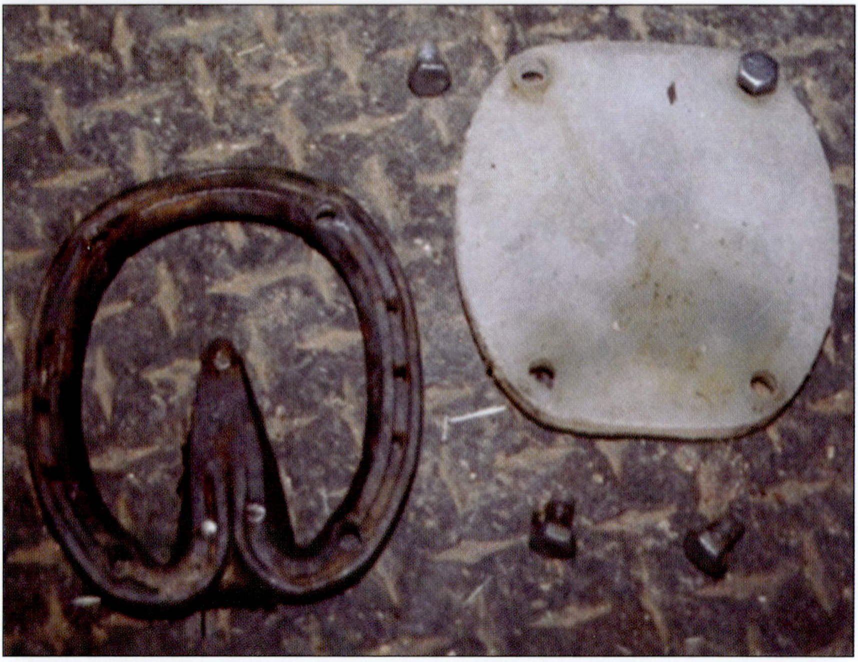

Figure 8-3. *Heart bar shoe with hospital plate made from 1/4″ copolymer plastic. © 2004 Doug Butler Enterprises, Inc. Used by permission.*

The edges of the frog must be visible on both sides and in front of the bar to prevent constriction of the paracuneal artery that runs down both sides of the frog. The exact position of the apex of the heart bar shoe is determined from measurements on lateral radiographs. Dr. Platt and Mr. Chapman have determined by experimentation that this position is at least 37 percent of the length of the distal phalanx bone behind its tip. A perpendicular line dropped from the dorsal edge at the base of the extensor process will also work. (See D. and J. Butler. *The Principles of Horseshoeing - P3*, page 555.).

The web (width) of the shoe must be narrow to prevent pressure on the circumflex artery. The foot surface of the shoe should be seated out. A rim pad may be needed to prevent sole pressure if the sole is flat or dropped. A hospital plate (removable ground surfacc pad) may be necessary when the sole is thin or the tip of the distal phalanx bone is exposed. A rolled-toe or rocker-toe is often useful as the horse will eventually wear the shoe to this configuration.

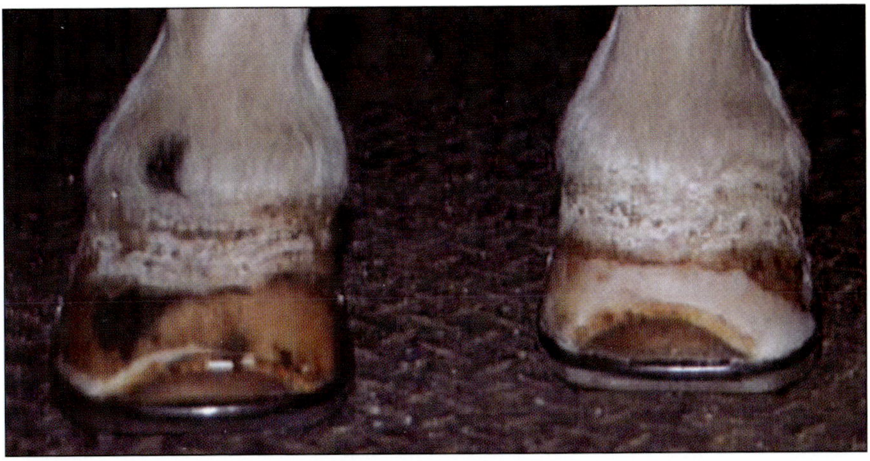

Figure 8-4. *Limited resection of hoof wall to drain abscesses. © 2004 Doug Butler Enterprises, Inc. Used by permission.*

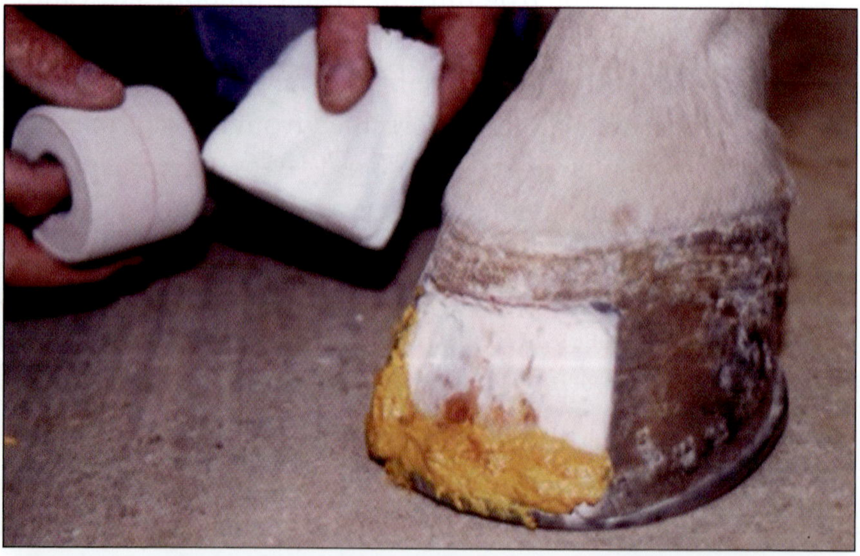

Figure 8-5. *Extensive resection of dorsal hoof wall to drain abscesses and allow normal hoof growth of wall. Photo © Doug Butler Enterprises, Inc. Used by permission.*

Dorsal hoof wall resection may be necessary

After the shoe is nailed in place and the clinches are finished, the front of the hoof wall can be resected (removed) down to the soft insensitive laminae. Resections relieve fluid pressure under the laminar wedge (scar horn) and help restore the blood supply to the front of the compressed coronary band.

Only hoof tissue is removed. There is no invasion of sensitive structures. This technique has the greatest chance of success if the heart bar or frog support shoes are applied early in the course of the disease.

Abscesses and seromas (serum pockets) that form due to lack of circulation caused by swelling are best drained from the front. Those drained from the bottom through the sole often develop painful exuberant granulation tissue.

Heart bar shoes must be reset frequently

Heart bar shoes must be reset frequently, at least every four weeks, to maintain bone column angle, shoe position and frog support. A long-term commitment to the horse's recovery is required. Most cases require therapeutic shoeing for at least six months. Some horses will require heart bars all their lives; a few will never be completely sound.

The heart bar shoe must be used without phenylbutazone (Bute). Painkillers such as Bute and Banamine cause the horse to further damage its feet by allowing it to stand and walk when it should be lying down. Bute also damages the gut and causes blood vessels to become more leaky. The damage caused by its use at the beginning may not become evident until later. Also, long-term use of Bute is said to inhibit thyroid gland function.

Foundered horses must be encouraged to lie down by providing a deep bed of shavings or straw. They must have expert nursing care and should be fed a nutritional supplement that will address their hormone imbalance like Farrier's Formula®.

Heart bar shoes are our most effective mechanical treatment tool

The heart bar shoe is the most effective tool we have to mechanically treat feet when laminar damage is present. Its effectiveness is due to its accommodation of the vascular anatomy of the foot. We must learn when to use it and how to

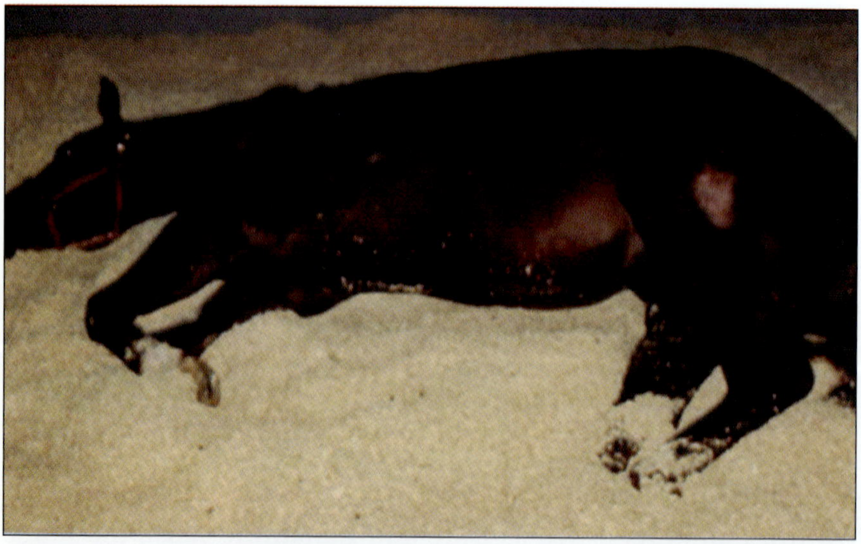

Figure 8-6. *Severely foundered horse in a deep-bedded stall. Note the decubitus ulcer on the hip. Photo © 2004 Doug Butler Enterprises, Inc. Used by permission.*

fit it. Today, we can choose from handmade, ready-made, flame-cut, welded, or aluminum shoes styles. Yet all must be fit with precision.

Some have passed judgment on the heart bar shoe by saying it doesn't work. Dr. D. Butler found that he had to shoe over 100 horses with these shoes before he felt confident in fitting them. Often, those who have trouble have had little or no experience making and fitting the shoe. In some cases, they haven't even shod 100 horses! Go to a specialist!

Refer difficult cases to specialists

General practitioner farriers should refer difficult founder cases to specialists who enjoy the challenging work and are experienced in helping horses with this life-threatening disease. Even the most experienced practitioners will not always be successful. It may take half a day to shoe a horse with precision-fit frog support shoes. Follow-up work is often required. Farriers must charge accordingly. Founder treatment is often long term and can be very expensive for the owner. Owners must understand the reasons for these precision mechanical treatment shoes and be committed to long-term care before treatment begins.

Conclusion

Laminitis and founder are very serious conditions, and it is important to use sound, time-tested mechanical as well as medical treatment regimens to treat them. While horses treated with more attention to detail have a greater chance of recovery, you must realize that no matter how treated, some horses simply will not recover.

The equine professional must become the horse owner's ally when treating laminitis and founder in order to have the greatest chance for a successful outcome. It is important that farriers, veterinarians and horse owners work together for the good of the horse; however, ultimately, the horse owner must make the final decision as to what is best for their horse.

In order to choose the most effective treatment regimen for laminitis and founder, you must know the predisposing cause, stage of the disease, mode of action and how best to prevent future attacks. The cause must be determined and removed or neutralized. The swelling or mode of action must be reduced to prevent further damage to the sensitive foot tissues. The damaged structures must be supported so the body can repair them. And finally, the destroyed tissue must be rebuilt by feeding an especially formulated feed supplement to encourage new hoof growth.

A Quick Guide to Basic Treatment Principles for Laminitis and Founder

---

1. **Veterinarian determines the cause and stage of the disease.**
   a. Get a complete history from the horse's caretaker(s).
   b. Observe the animal in its environment.
   c. Run diagnostic blood test(s).
   d. Take radiographs to reveal bone remodeling and position.
   e. Discuss prognosis and explore options with client, including euthanasia.

2. **Veterinarian treats the cause of the acute systemic disease medically.**
   a. Treat laminitis as an emergency! Object is to reduce pressure inside hoof capsule.
   b. Soak the feet in ice cold water mixed with Epsom salts to prevent or reduce inflammation.
   c. Administer mineral oil by stomach tube to evacuate the gut.
   d. Give a powerful blood vessel contractor such as Ergonovine.
   e. Use an anti-inflammatory that doesn't sedate, such as Dipyrone.
   f. Do not give long-term pain medications such as Bute or Banamine.
   g. Apply DMSO topically below the fetlock to reduce swelling.

h. Consider giving DMSO with Dextrose in the vein to get fluid out of tissues.

i. Relax superficial and deep flexor muscles with Robaxin. Don't do tenotomy!

j. Give Eq Stim to boost system immunity and prevent osteomyelitis.

k. Give Baytril or Ampicillin and Gentomycin I.V. if infection is present.

l. Lasix will help pull salt out of the tissues.

3. Veterinarian takes consistent, measurable radiographs.

a. Place markers on the hoof by using a wire or nail on toe, thumb tack on frog.

b. Take radiographs at a consistent distance or correct for magnification.

c. Look for evidence of bone remodeling.

d. Calculate the position of the apex of shoe frog support. 37 percent of DP bone base.

4. Farrier trims hoof and constructs or chooses shoes according to radiograph.

a. Trim hoof to align pastern axis. This usually means lowering the heels and cutting back the toe.

b. Dress the toe back so it is parallel with the dorsal surface of the coffin bone.

c. Trim the frog so it is soft and level.

d. Use creased shoe so can pull nails without injuring sole.

5. Farrier fits accurate heart bar shoes for mechanical support.

a. Fit the shoe around the DP bone circumference.

b. Adjust bar length to fit as marked.

c. Form bar to frog shape. Fit bar so can see frog all around including point of frog.

d. Build up frog support with leather or plastic shims or soft composite to get level.

e. Make a hospital or treatment plate, if sole is perforated or sore.

6. Farrier applies shoes and "reads" the horse.

a. Feel and adjust pressure when frog is squeezed and spreads in every direction.

b. "Read" the horse to determine its response to applied frog pressure.

c. Place nails behind point of bar. Leave rough clinches to rasp off at reset.

d. Remove excess hoof after nailing.

e. Resect dorsal wall to drain abscesses and seromas under direction of vet.

f. Use Sugardine or Magna Paste to poultice abscesses and prevent infection.

g. Bandage resected area with antiseptic until laminae harden.

7. **Owner must monitor the horse daily; the farrier must reset the shoes monthly; and the veterinarian must drain abscesses and periodically monitor the horse's nutritional condition.**
   a. Provide a deep bed (18 inches) so horse will lie down to prevent further damage.
   b. Keep the feet clean — change dressings at least every other day.
   c. Schedule regular farrier and veterinarian visits and monthly resets.
   d. Feed Farrier's Formula® supplement to aid healing and treat hormone imbalance.

Remember!

Prevention of laminitis is more successful than treatment!

About the Authors and Contributors

Doug Butler, PhD, CJF, FWCF, is the principal author of *The Principles of Horseshoeing (P3)*, the most widely used farrier textbook in the world. He has been using heart bar shoes for over 22 years to mechanically treat laminitis/founder. He won the North American Challenge Cup Horseshoeing Competition in 1980 and the Heart Bar Shoe Making Contest at the AFA Convention in 1985 and 1986. From his business, Butler Professional Farrier School, LLC, 495 Table Rd., Crawford, Nebraska 69339, 1-800-728-3826, he shoes and rehabilitates difficult founder cases, consults, publishes, speaks, and presents the annual Farrier Focus® Business Conference. **www.farrierfocus.com.** E-mail doug@dougbutler.com

Frank Gravlee, DVM, MS, CNS, is the founder of Life Data Labs, Inc., P.O. Box 349, 12290 Hwy. 72, Cherokee, Alabama 35616, 1-800-624-1873. He developed Farrier's Formula® feed supplement 22 years ago. His frequently copied but never equaled formula is used world-wide and has saved the lives of many horses. His manufacturing plant where the pelleted supplement is manufactured is ISO certified. All Life Data products are manufactured to the highest standards. New products are invented and tested in a state-of-the-art laboratory and on a research farm. Dr. Gravlee has developed methods of medically treating founder that have a high degree of success. **www.lifedatalabs.com.** E-mail jfgravlee@lifedatalabs.com.

George Platt, DVM, and **Burney Chapman,** CJF (deceased), conceived the idea of using the heart bar or frog support shoe to mechanically treat laminitis and founder in this generation. They first presented their findings at the American Association of Equine practitioners in 1984. Their ideas have been frequently copied and other ideas have been tried, yet their techniques are still the most consistently successful way to mechanically treat this devastating disease of horses.

21 Questions to Test Your Knowledge of Laminitis and Founder

1. Laminitis is:
   a. a systemic disease that starts as inflammation in the foot.
   b. a local disease between the hoof and bones within it.
   c. a systemic disease that results in the sinking of the bone column in the hoof.
   d. more deadly than founder to heavy horses.
2. Founder is:
   a. the same as laminitis.
   b. a sinking or rotation of the coffin bone within the hoof.
   c. less serious than laminitis.
   d. a systemic disease caused by a virus in the feed.
3. Fructans are:
   a. plant sugars that are at the highest levels in spring in the early morning.
   b. plant proteins that are at their highest levels in spring in late afternoon.
   c. plant carbohydrates thought to be a key trigger of laminitis.
   d. produced at their highest levels by pasture plants with dew on them.
4. Bedding that may cause laminitis:
   a. yellow pine shavings.
   b. white oak shavings.
   c. black walnut shavings.
   d. maple sawdust.
5. The object of frog support shoeing is to:
   a. push the coffin bone back into position in the foot.
   b. stabilize and support the bone so the horse can grow a new hoof.
   c. force the blood back into the toe of the hoof to heal the bone.
   d. relieve pressure from the diseased heel by shifting weight to the healthy frog.

6. Sole support shoeing:
   a. restores circulation to the circumflex artery.
   b. pushes the coffin bone back in place.
   c. can compress the vessels of the solar corium and cause abscesses.
   d. is consistently more effective than frog support shoeing.
7. Concussion induced founder is usually a condition of horses:
   a. with weak laminae and sustained work on a hard surface.
   b. with studs or borium that are trotted across a road.
   c. that are shod with clips that are hammered in.
   d. that occasionally jump high obstacles barefoot.
8. Founder can be caused by:
   a. allergic reactions to drugs, vaccines or dewormers.
   b. temperature changes.
   c. environmental changes.
   d. any of the above.
9. Conditions that do not put a horse at risk for laminitis:
   a. obesity, bloodlines, poor farriery.
   b. systemic infection, obesity, colic.
   c. mud, running with the herd, timothy hay.
   d. alfalfa pasture, clover hay, fat in the grain ration.
10. Plants that should not be grazed in any amount by horses:
    a. alfalfa, clover, birdsfoot trefoil.
    b. maple leaves, yew bush, jimson weed.
    c. b and d.
    d. senecio, astralagus, larkspur.
11. Early detection of laminitis is difficult because:
    a. there is no obvious change in skin color.
    b. blood samples take a long time to analyze.
    c. horses can't talk and show us where it hurts.
    d. horses are rarely lame until the tissues in the foot are affected.

12. Identifying the cause of laminitis is necessary to:
    a. prevent your other horses from getting the disease.
    b. change how the mechanical treatment is done.
    c. change how the medical treatment is done.
    d. make you a better horseman.

13. Horses that have had laminitis before are:
    a. are immunized and can't get it again.
    b. likely to have a less serious case if they get it again.
    c. are at increased risk to get it again.
    d. should be fed a high fat ration.

14. Older horses with Cushing's disease or pituitary tumors:
    a. should be fed with younger horses.
    b. should be fed individually a feed supplement to assist hormone balance.
    c. should be fed a Bute supplement.
    d. should always be shod with open shoes.

15. As soon as laminitis is suspected:
    a. call the vet to obtain diagnosis and first medical therapy.
    b. call the farrier to fit shoes or trim with frog support.
    c. stand the horse in ice water.
    d. all of the above.

16. To prevent laminitis:
    a. secure feed in a room not accessible to loose horses.
    b. turn out horses on lush pasture only on sunny days.
    c. avoid feeding low nutrient quality hay.
    d. provide fresh water.

17. Signs of laminitis may include:
    a. strong digital pulses, standing back on the front feet.
    b. reluctance to walk, laying down more than usual.
    c. sweating, elevated respiration, slight fever.
    d. any of the above.

18. To prevent laminitis:
    a. spray pastures for weeds.
    b. avoid overfeeding idle horses by muzzling or drylotting.
    c. keep the horse barefoot.
    d. feed garlic supplement.

19. Ask prospective health care providers:
    a. what school did you attend?
    b. have you ever owned a horse?
    c. who (farrier or vet) do you work with on laminitis cases?
    d. are you certified and experienced in therapeutic work?

20. This percentage of horses completely recover from laminitis in the U. S.:
    a. 93
    b. 74
    c. 55
    d. 36

21. Bute should not be used as a long-term treatment for laminitis because:
    a. it causes cecal ulcers.
    b. it causes an increase in appetite.
    c. it causes further damage to the laminae.
    d. it causes loose shoes

KEY: 1 - a; 2 - b; 3 - c; 4 - c; 5 - b; 6 - c; 7 - a; 8 - d; 9 - c; 10 - c; 11 - d; 12 - a; 13 - c; 14 - b; 15 - d; 16 - a; 17 - d; 18 - b; 19 - c; 20 - b; 21 - c.